Medicines:
Responsible Prescribing

Editor:
F. O. Wells

Executive Editors:
P. F. D'Arcy and D. W. G. Harron

MEDICINES:
RESPONSIBLE PRESCRIBING

Edited by:

F. O. Wells, MB BS, MFPM,
Director, Medical Affairs,
Association of the British Pharmaceutical Association

Executive Editors:

P. F. D'Arcy, OBE, BPharm, PhD, DSc, FRPharmS, FRSC, FPSNI
Professor of Pharmacy in The Queen's University of Belfast

D. W. G. Harron, BSc, PhD, FRPharmS, MPSNI
Reader in Pharmacology, Department of Therapeutics and Pharmacology,
The Queen's University of Belfast

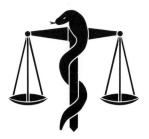

Published at The Queen's University of Belfast

British Library Cataloguing in Publication Data

Medicines: Responsible Prescribing
    Wells, F. O. (Editor)
    D'Arcy, P. F. and Harron, D. W. G. (Executive Editors)

ISBN 0 85389 416 7

Distributed by Greystone Books Ltd.,
Caulside Drive,
Antrim, N. Ireland.

Typeset by W. & G. Baird Ltd.
Printed in Northern Ireland by W. & G. Baird Ltd.

To Catherine and Henrietta

Acknowledgements

My grateful thanks are due to all the contributors who responded, without exception, so willingly to my request that they might write a chapter. My thanks are also due in great measure to my executive editors, Dean Harron and Pat D'Arcy, with whom, as before, it has been a great stimulus to work. Those thanks must also be extended to the whole team at The Queen's University of Belfast publication and printing departments, who have been responsible for producing a top quality book, which is pleasing to handle.

My greatest thanks are due to my long-suffering, over-worked secretary Lesley Hines, who has had to put up with the effects of the stresses and strains which any editor is bound to experience. Because of the co-operation of everyone mentioned above, these stresses and strains have been kept to an absolute minimum, which I greatly appreciate.

Whitehall, London   Frank Wells
January 1992

Foreword

by

Lord Walton of Detchant

It is a pleasure to welcome the publication of this volume, which has been skillfully edited by my friend Dr Frank Wells, Director of Medical Affairs for the Association of the British Pharmaceutical Industry (APBI). While its publication has been sponsored by the ABPI, the chapters which follow have almost all been written by persons who have no direct association with the industry. Nevertheless, the attitude of that industry towards the indicative prescribing scheme for general practitioners is now regarded by politicians, doctors and managers alike to be generally responsible. The message enshrined in this book throughout is, as Dr Wells himself once said, timeless; it is that prescribing should always be responsible.

Since I graduated in medicine more than 45 years ago I and all those of my generation have witnessed a veritable pharmacological revolution. Even in my own specialty of neurology, once regarded by many as being solely a descriptive and diagnostic art, the management of many diseases such as epilepsy and parkinsonism, to quote but two examples, has been transformed by the introduction of new remedies so designed as to offer logically and soundly based treatment made possible through the fruits of fundamental laboratory research. There can be no disputing the fact that many drugs now available across the whole field of medicine have specific and clearly defined indications and have made remarkable contributions to patient care. The conquest of many infections, too, has been made possible by the introduction of generations of new antibiotics which have fortunately become available at a time when resistance to some of the earlier remedies has become widespread. In cardiovascular disease, in chemotherapy for malignant disease and in many autoimmune disorders which can now effectively be controlled by steroids, we have seen many other major advances. But among these new drugs are many potent remedies with real and potential side-effects, even in a limited number of patients, so that they, like the immensely powerful psychotropic agents now at the disposal of the medical profession, have to be handled carefully and judiciously. Hence the responsibility of the prescribing doctor has become truly awesome. Not only must he or she be aware of the risks as well as the benefits of the medication to be prescribed, but another major component, namely that of cost and cost-effectiveness, has had to be introduced into the therapeutic equation not just in the United Kingdom but throughout the developed world where the rising burden of health costs has given concern to governments and other providers alike. Education, therefore, in the proper and responsible use of drugs has never been more vital than it is today and I believe that this book will prove to be a comprehensive and authoritative guide. Carefully and judiciously planned, well edited, and written by acknowledged experts, it will repay careful study by all doctors and is likely in my opinion to make a major contribution to responsible prescribing.

John Walton
Oxford
January 1992

Introduction

During the past two years, the Association of the British Pharmaceutical Industry has been closely associated with the various activities which arose from the publication of two documents from the Department of Health on Improving Prescribing. The whole thrust of these activities has been concentrated on the effectiveness of medicines used appropriately in the delivery of patient care – in other words, Responsible Prescribing.

This book encapsulates many of these activities, written as it is by a series of authors who are all, in their different ways, important players in the field of prescribing. Jane Richards and Linda Stone are in the forward line, prescribing and dispensing to patients. Mahendra Mashru and Alastair Hepburn are advisers on prescribing, and Gordon England supports them. Geoffrey Podger is, as he describes himself, a mandarin, responsible for ensuring that the current UK Government policy on prescribing in our National Health Service is intelligible. Colin Hitchings, in the light of that policy, oversees the pharmaceutical service of an NHS region. Douglas Ball makes data available about prescribing, Conrad Harris helps doctors to use that data effectively, and Nick Hough provides more information through the Medicines Resource Centre. Sandy Florence teaches about medicines, as does Philip Reilly who is also in the forward line as a prescriber. Michael Orme teaches, too, and is familiar with both hospital and general practitioner prescribing. George Teeling Smith, Peter Lumley and I operate from within the industry, which actually produces the medicines to be prescribed.

Although much of the book revolves around the Indicative Prescribing Scheme, introduced into the United Kingdom on 1 April 1991, the principles of responsible prescribing are timeless, and I hope readers from outside these shores will derive information which is of some value, as well as interest, from the various chapters. Nevertheless, it is for general practitioners, and the relevant levels of NHS health management that this book is primarily intended. My colleagues in the pharmaceutical industry will, I hope, also derive a great deal of information from it.

Frank Wells
January 1992

Contributors

Ball, D. G., MBCS
Director of Information Technology, Prescription Pricing Authority.

England, A. G., BSc, MISC, MB, ChB
Director, Medical Advisers Support Centre.

Florence, A. T., DSc, FRSC, FRSE, FRPharmS
Dean, School of Pharmacy, University of London.

Harris, C. M., MEd, MB, ChB, FRCGP, DObstRCOG
Director, Prescribing Research Unit (Department of General Practice), University of Leeds.

Hepburn, A., MSc, MB, BS, MRCGP
Consultant Adviser in Primary Care, North West Thames and South West Thames Regional Health Authorities.

Hitchings, C. R., BPharm, MSc, FRPharmS, MCPP
Regional Pharmaceutical Officer, South West Thames Regional Health Authority.

Hough, N., MSc, MRPharmS
Director, Medicines Resource Centre.

Lumley, P. F., MIPR
Director of Public Affairs, The Association of the British Pharmaceutical Industry.

Mashru, M. K., MD, MB, MChir, MRCS, LRCP, LMSSA, MRCGP
Medical Adviser, Brent and Harrow Family Health Services Authority.

Orme, M. C. L'E., MA, MD, FRCP, FFPM
Dean, Faculty of Medicine and Professor of Pharmacology and Therapeutics, University of Liverpool.

Podger, G. J. F., MA (Oxon)
Assistant Secretary, Department of Health.

Reilly, P. M., MD, MB, BCh, BAO, FRCGP
Head of Department of General Practice, Queen's University of Belfast.

Richards, S. J., MB, BS, MRCS, LRCP, FRCGP, DObstRCOG, DCH
General Practitioner, Exeter.

Teeling Smith, G., OBE, BA, FRPharmS
Director, Office of Health Economics.

Stone, L., BPharmS, MRPharmS
Community Pharmacist, Past President, Royal Pharmaceutical Society of Great Britain.

Wells, F. O., MB, BS, MFPM
Director of Medical Affairs, The Association of the British Pharmaceutical Industry.

Biographical Details of the Contributors

Douglas Ball managed a transport business prior to his career in computing, which spans a period of twenty one years. It began with Northern Ireland Electricity, where he was responsible for the development of financial and engineering systems, development systems, and the training of computing staff. After seven years, he moved to the Prescription Pricing Authority, where, as Director of Information Technology at the PPA, he is responsible for all of the Authority's computing systems, the Contractors Payment System, the generation of PACT data, and the involvement of the PPA in the Indicative Prescribing Scheme.

Gordon England before taking up medicine, qualified in physics and engineering and worked as a research hydrodynamicist in the aircraft industry. After a clinical career, which included research fellowships in cardiology and renal medicine, he became Scientific Adviser to the Mersey Regional Health Authority. He holds an Honorary Lectureship in the Department of Public Health Medicine at the University of Liverpool, and his research interests include the use of expert systems in clinical medicine, the epidemiology of heart disease, and prescribing protocols. In 1990 he was appointed Director of the Medical Advisers Support Centre.

Alexander Florence is Dean of the School of Pharmacy of the University of London, and was, until 1989, Professor of Pharmaceutics at the University of Strathclyde. Since 1972 he has been involved with medicines regulation in the UK, and is a member of the Committee on Safety of Medicines and Chairman of its Sub-committee on Chemistry, Pharmacy and Standards. His research interests focus on drug delivery and targeting. He is the author or co-author of a number of textbooks, including the Physiochemical Principles of Pharmacy; and Surfactant Systems. He is the editor of Volumes 1 and 2 of Topics of Pharmacy.

Conrad Harris practised for twelve years on Merseyside before starting an academic career which led him, through Manchester and London, to a chair in the Department of General Practice in the University of Leeds. He has been involved in prescribing research for twelve years, and for several years was a member of the Prescription Pricing Authority, helping to create PACT. He has co-authored a book on analysis of prescribing which was distributed to every practice in England, and since 1990 has been the Director of the Prescribing Research Unit in Leeds University.

Alastair Hepburn held hospital posts in Eastbourne and Glasgow before becoming a principal in general practice in North West Durham, where he practised for fifteen years. During that time he held part-time posts as Hospital Practitioner in Geriatrics, and Tutor in Family Medicine at the University of Newcastle. He then became Senior Medical Officer to the Department of Health, and in 1990 commenced his post as Consultant Adviser in Primary Care, with particular responsibilities for prescribing, in the North West Thames and South West Thames Regions.

Colin Hitchings qualified in pharmacy at the University of Nottingham in 1963, and after a distinguished career in various pharmacy fields in 1981 he became Regional Pharmaceutical Officer to the South West Thames Regional Health Authority. He was President of the Royal Pharmaceutical Society of Great Britain in 1983–84, and has served on its Council for many years before and since. He has been President of the International Pharmaceutical Federation, and of the Guild of Hospital Pharmacists, and since 1978 he has been a member (and since 1989 Deputy Chairman) of the Joint Formulary Committee, responsible for producing the British National Formulary.

Nicholas Hough qualified in 1981 and was employed as a hospital pharmacist for five years, during which time he undertook an MSc in Clinical Pharmacology; at the same time he held the post of teacher/practitioner in conjunction with the School of Pharmacy at Portsmouth Polytechnic. He then joined the International Drug Surveillance Department of Glaxo Group Research for three years, as principal clinical research scientist before taking up his present position as Director of the Medicines Resource Centre.

Peter Lumley, who began his career as a local newspaper journalist, joined Glaxo Laboratories at Greenford in 1964 where he was appointed Public Affairs Manager in 1971. He joined the association of the British Pharmaceutical Industry in 1973 as Information Services Manager and was appointed Director of Public Affairs in May 1989, with responsibility for the Association's parliamentary and media relations activities, publications, advertising and member company communication.

Mahendra Mashru qualified from Cambridge in 1981, and after hous appointments at Addenbrookes Hospital became a vocational trainee in general practice in Hillingdon. Since 1985 he has been a principal in general pracice in Ruislip, which he now fulfils on a part-time basis. He is a GP tutor at Hillingdon Hospital, has a masters degree in general practice from the University of London, and since 1990 has been Medical Director of the Brent and Harrow Family Health Services Authority.

Michael Orme studied at Cambridge University and Kings College Hospital, London. Thereafter he trained at the Hammersmith, Brompton and St. Mary's Hospitals in London in General Medicine, before returning to Hammersmith Hospital in 1968 with an MRC training fellowship in Clinical Pharmacology. He then worked for eighteen months at the Karolinska Institute in Stockholm during 1973 and 1974, following which in 1975 he was appointed Senior Lecturer in Clinical Pharmacology at Liverpool. He was promoted to Reader in 1981, and to a personal chair in 1984 which he still holds. He is also currently Dean of the Faculty of Medicine at the University of Liverpool.

Geoffrey Podger is a career civil servant who joined the then Department of Health in 1982, having previously worked for the Ministry of Defence and the North Atlantic Treaty Organisation. In 1985 he became Secretary to the NHS Management Board and Private Secretary to its Chairman and Chief Executive. This was followed by two years as Principal Private Secretary to the Secretary of State for Social Services, and he is now Project Manager for both the GP Funding Initiative and the Indicative Prescribing Scheme.

Philip Reilly is a graduate of Queen's University, Belfast, and for many years has been a general practitioner. Since 1978 he has been Senior Lecturer in

General Practice until 1990 when he was granted the Chair of General Practice at Queen's University, Belfast. He was the UK Prescribing Fellow of the Royal College of General Practitioners from 1987 to 1990, and he will be a member of the UK Medicines Commission for four years, commencing in January 1992.

Jane Richards was brought up and educated in Crediton, Devon, and trained at University College and Hospital in London. After hospital experience in Plymouth, she joined a rural dispensing practice in Gloucestershire, and since 1965 has been a principal in a large health centre general practice in Exeter. She has been a member of the Council of the British Medical Association since 1971, and of the General Medical Services Committee since 1978. She has been the Chairman of the GMSC Prescribing Sub-committee since its inception, is a member of the Prescription Pricing Authority, and a member of the Advisory Committee on NHS Drugs. She was recently appointed to the Joint Formulary Committee, responsible for the British National Formulary.

George Teeling Smith took an honours degree in mathematics and natural sciences at Cambridge, before qualifying as a pharmacist in Edinburgh. After ten years in the pharmaceutical industry in 1962 he was appointed as the founder Director of the Office of Health Economics, a post which he still holds. Since 1980 he has also been Professor Associate in Health Economics at Brunel University, and he has written and lectured extensively on the economics of medical care and the pharmaceutical industry.

Linda Stone is a second generation community pharmacist, who most recently has served from 1990 to 1991 as President of the Royal Pharmaceutical Society of Great Britain. Prior to that she was Chairman and a Member of various Committees of the Royal Pharmaceutical Society, including Chairman, in 1989/90, of its Working Party on Labelling. Since 1989 she has been Chairman of the Royal Society for the Prevention of Accidents, and, since 1987, of its Home and Leisure Safety Committee.

Frank Wells graduated from the Royal London Hospital, and after two years experience in hospital appointments became a general practitioner in Ipswich, Suffolk, where he was in practice for nearly twenty years. In 1979 he was appointed Under Secretary of the British Medical Association, of the Council of which he is now an elected member. In 1986 he became Director of Medical Affairs of the Association of the British Pharmaceutical Industry, where he is responsible for servicing the Medical Committee and associated sub-committees and working parties, and for providing an interface between the medical profession and the pharmaceutical industry.

Contents

1   Practical Aspects of Responsible General Practitioner Prescribing

Jane Richards

GP Prescribing

Prescribing by general practitioners has been under critical scrutiny for decades. Many people both in and outside the profession think that they know more about it than GPs do themselves. They certainly subtend a substantial amount of the overall NHS bill – £2.43 billion for England alone in 1989–90 – and therefore have to be accountable to the government for what they do. They are also subject to scrutiny from other sources every time they pick up their pens and FP 10s to prescribe. Primarily, however, they are accountable to their patients for what and how they prescribe but they also come under pressure from the pharmaceutical industry, the hospital service and their pharmacist colleagues. Now in addition they have to 'answer sufficiently' any queries from the Medical Adviser to their contracting Family Health Service Authority (FHSA). So in this context, what is good prescribing?

The General Medical Services Committee of the BMA has long held the view that good prescribing is both rational and cost-effective. The government would wish doctors to concentrate on the second aspect and in order to facilitate this has developed both PACT and, more recently, the Indicative Prescribing Scheme. It therefore appears to general practitioners that where the Department of Health is concerned good prescribing is not just value for money but better value for less money. The government has, however, clearly stated that patients will get all the medicines that they need including high cost items when these are required, and this must not be forgotten.

PACT – Prescribing Analysis and Cost – has already had an impact on the pattern and price of drug provision by providing GPs with data on what they have actually prescribed and at what cost, as distinct from what they thought they had done. This is described and discussed elsewhere in this book as is the Indicative Prescribing Scheme which depends upon the same data base, captured by the Prescription Pricing Authority as part of the process of paying pharmacists. General practitioners are now all able to be fully aware of the costs of their own prescribing and how these relate to those of their colleagues both locally and nationally, but neither of these information systems tell them whether their prescribing is effective or rational. Apart from the actual number of patients registered with them, there is no correlation with patient care.

There are other very important factors which contribute to rational effective prescribing; these include the pharmacology and clinical efficacy, safety and appropriateness of the medication and whether patients comply with how they have been told to take it. Let us look at prescribing through the eyes and interests of those groups mentioned earlier on.

Patients

Patients come first. They are critical of 'profligacy' in public debate when it relates to others, until their own needs – or wants – come into the frame. Then the debate changes, and general practitioners are under pressure to prescribe when that is what the patient perceives as being appropriate. This is an area which, when they talk of 'needs', the politicians are probably excluding: strictly scientifically there may well not be a 'need' for medication for certain conditions, but the overall continuing care of the patient in which GPs are so closely involved does require a 'prescription'. The credo of the current government is 'market forces' and the general practitioner's contract has been drawn up in this mode. GPs believe that, if they do not respond is some way to the perceived needs of their patients, they will certainly suffer in the market place of competition for them. Sadly more patients means less time with each, so less time to explain why no medication is indicated in certain circumstances; it is easier to reach for the pad and the prescribed placebo. In addition, the increased proportion of the income of general practitioners which is received from capitation fees has greatly hazarded the progress of the education of their patients that there is not a 'pill for every ill', and that the pen is not mightier than the word. Patient education on the need or otherwise for medication is an important aspect of responsible prescribing.

Prescription Charges

Frequent and significant increases in prescription charges are another cause of pressure by patients on their GPs to prescribe less than sensibly, though the charge only applies to about 20% of prescriptions. It cannot be said that it is irrational to prescribe for three months at a time, nor is it extravagant or uneconomical if the patient is on long term medication, well stabilised and compliant, and is being appropriately monitored, but there is potential for waste and 'use by' dates might be exceeded. It is accepted for pill prescribing and perhaps hormone replacement therapy (HRT), but for little else. Understandably community pharmacists do not like it as it reduces their fee income, but some patients who have difficulty getting their prescriptions made up, particularly in country areas, definitely do like it. Hopefully FHSAs and their advisers will continue to allow flexibility in this area while prescribers continue to recognise that repeat prescriptions should normally be for one month's supply.

Repeat prescribing is another area of contention. It is not of itself a sin but it does need to be carefully controlled by the prescribing doctor. Rigid protocols are not the answer; periodicity of monitoring has to be determined for the individual patient as well as for the condition being treated. Periodicity of prescribing can have a different pattern so long as the arangements for both monitoring and prescribing are agreed and understood by the patient, the doctor and the doctor's staff from the outset. The records of drugs allowed as repeats must be clear and unequivocal.

It is responsible prescribing policy to look critically at the length of short courses of treatment, of such medicines as antibiotics, and to choose the optimum for each patient rather than a standard course which may be wastefully long or equally wastefully inadequate.

However correct the drug is for the condition and however cost-effective in theory it is not good prescribing if patients cannot or do not comply with the regime defined. Exploring such factors as whether patients remember doses better three times a day or only once is therefore time well spent. That they understand how medication should be taken is part of the prescribing process and should not be left solely to the pharmacist. Rational prescribing in the interests of good patient care is therefore at times a negotiated compromise to achieve compliance.

Over- and Underprescribing

All can agree that there is sometimes overprescribing. The amount of medicines returned in DUMP campaigns are a measure of that. All GPs have probably overprescribed at some time, and they all need to exercise constant vigilance in their prescribing for elderly people who live alone. Recently, I found a cache of tablets in the chest of drawers of an old lady whose insidiously increasing dementia had masked her poor compliance. Invading her privacy in order to discover such a problem is a delicate matter and one each doctor has to work out how best to handle.

All can also agree that there is sometimes underprescribing. Some of this is due to unawareness of the existence of treatment for certain conditions, some is due to under-diagnosis of treatable conditions, and some is undoubtedly as a reaction to the pressures on GPs to curtail prescribing costs.

Budgets

Two potentially conflicting aspects of the provision of medicines must be mentioned, involving as they do the FHSA and the hospital service. As clearly set out in a later chapter, the Regional Health Authority (RHA) has a firm drug budget and is responsible for prescribing policies adopted throughout the region. It gives the FHSA its firm budget and oversees the hospital prescribing but the District Health Authorities and the NHS Trust hospitals determine their own actual drug budgets. The FHSA has to square the circle of GP prescribing, for it is at that level that the resolution between firm and indicative or 'top down' and 'bottom up' takes place. Any spare money in the RHA disbursement to the FHSA may be needed for unanticipated in-year increases by practices and any expansion of the pharmaceutical services themselves. The hospitals do not have the same flexibility and still see the budget for general practitioner prescribing as open-ended; the problems of the transfer of hospital prescribing costs to GPs have not yet been solved. That is a price we have had to pay for the FPS drug budget not being cash-limited and I do not see the FHSA facilitated discussions between GPs and hospital doctors being any more successful than previous ones until the government publishes the recommendations of its national working party on this subject.

Hospital prescribing does have a marked influence on local general practitioner prescribing quite apart from transfer or 'cost shifting'. However GPs are not bound to prescribe what a consultant recommends regardless, as they have to take full clinical and legal responsibility for every prescription they sign. Today they take economic responsibility also. If a consultant continues to carry clinical responsibility for the care of the patient, he should continue to prescribe for that element for which he is responsible. When a consultant returns the care of the patient to the general practitioner and recommends a particular new medication the GP must familiarise himself with all the relevant information about that medicine before continuing to prescribe it; and there are potential problems when a patient who is taking part in a clinical trial on a new medicine is discharged from the hospital. The GP must be fully aware of what he is doing if he prescribes such a substance even on hospital recommendation, and both parties must be aware of the implications of prescribing an unlicensed medicine, or a licensed medicine for an unlicensed indication.

Formularies

Turning to formularies, those produced in hospitals are based on fulfilling clinical need and providing the most cost effective forms available to the hospital pharmacy and these may be more expensive in the community where such bulk purchasing contracts are not available. Most hospital prescribing and dispensing is generic which may be quite confusing to patients when discharged back into the community. Great care is needed to explain such differences in nomenclature and appearances when patients revert to GP prescribing. General practitioners need to influence their hospital colleagues not to change their patients' medication for no better reason than that the particular drug used is not in their formulary; the GP might have had to choose it for very good clinical reasons. There should always be a general practitioner on a hospital Drug and Therapeutics Committee as many difficulties can be ironed out in this forum and misunderstandings corrected.

Good prescribing in the eyes of community pharmacists relates particularly to the mechanics of the prescription, whether it is correctly and clearly written to provide an unambiguous order with full instructions for the patient. Computer generated prescriptions can be an answer to the problems of legibility but not all printers are of an adequate quality and the programmes on some systems are poor. The Prescription Pricing Authority has some fearsome examples of what can go wrong both with quantities and doctor identifying numbers. The drug dictionaries of some systems are still inadequate, particularly in relation to appliances.

Compliance by patients is partly dependent upon the instructions they are given for the taking of the medication. If instructions are not included on the prescription form and it is up to the pharmacists to include the standard instructions on the label or even just 'as directed', it is not surprising that compliance is poor and treatment less than successful.

Pharmaceutical Industry

Lastly, I come to the pharmaceutical industry which would like general practitioners to be both innovative and conventional doctors at the same time, and prescribe their products both new and old. The drug firm representative has long been the GP's friend, providing information and goodies and educational opportunities. GPs do need to remember, though, that all they say is not gospel. They are a sales force, albeit with a very strict code of practice which the ABPI administers firmly. Because a drug is new it is not necessarily miraculous, but not is it irresponsible to prescribe it as some academics would have us believe. We must as ever use our clinical judgement. Various publications, including the *British National Formulary, Drug and Therapeutics Bulletin, Prescribers Notes* and local drug information pharmacists provide a great deal of objective information. Many Drug and Therapeutics Committees produce their own bulletins and the Medicines Resource Centre (MeReC) has started well with its publications. The *Data Sheet Compendium* published by the ABPI is a very valuable source of information.

At the end of the day, however, we must be grateful to our pharmaceutical industry in this country which continues to produce really new and useful drugs; it is innovative even if we are not and needs to be successful to maintain the research and development funds that allow it to be so. Good quality drugs come from a good quality industry.

Patients Come First

I commented early in this chapter that patients come first. I now come back to patients for they and their health are the object of the whole exercise of prescribing, not financial wizardry. Whatever happens in the next few years, with indicative budgets, medical advisers querying GP prescribing and, Europe altering the advertising and marketing of drugs after 1992, the ultimate consideration is the treatment of the individual patient. I believe that if general practitioners prescribe clinically correctly, rationally and with due respect for cost implications, which will include all other aspects of patient care and well-being, then they will be prescribing responsibly.

2　The Indicative Prescribing Scheme

Geoffrey Podger

Introduction

The origins of the Indicative Prescribing Scheme lie in the Government White Paper *Working for Patients* published in January 1989 which sets out the overall agenda of the NHS Reforms. Further amplification of the proposals was given in Working Paper 4 of the NHS Review series published in March 1989. There then followed a period of extensive consultation with outside interests including, in particular, representatives of the medical and pharmaceutical professions and of the pharmaceutical industry. The Indicative Prescribing Scheme was significantly further developed to reflect the outcome of this consultation process and the Government's definitive plans for implementing the Scheme were published in *Improving Prescribing* published in May 1990. The purpose of this Chapter is to describe the reasoning behind the scheme outlined in *Improving Prescribing*, how it will be implemented and what it is hoped to achieve.

Why Have the Scheme?

The simple answer to this very proper question is that given by the Rt Hon Kenneth Clarke QC MP when he was Secretary of State for Health. In a wide-ranging speech on the Government's approach to Family Health Service (FHS) prescribing delivered on 16 February 1990 Mr Clarke said 'This Government – again like any Government – has to recognise that it has a duty to patients to ensure that they do not suffer from inappropriate prescribing and to both the taxpayer and the NHS generally to ensure that we spend what we need to on necessary drugs – no more and no less.'

In the light of Mr Clarke's general observations, it is perhaps worth considering the inadequacies in the previous system which the Indicative Prescribing Scheme seeks to address. It should be said at the outset on quality of prescribing, as Mr Clarke did in his speech, that 'it is the medical profession itself which is taking the lead in examining the quality of prescribing and seeking to improve it still further. I applaud this unequivocally . . .'. Equally we do have to recognise that, hitherto, there has been a lack of a comprehensive framework within which to examine quality of prescribing by all practices and that this is an area where many professional studies have recognised that there is still room for improvement.

The cost of Family Health Service prescribing must be a matter for legitimate concern by Government. Over £2.1 billion was spent in England on FHS prescribing in 1990/91 before even taking account of the consequential cost of pharmacist remuneration. Moreover there has been a very high rate of growth in real terms with increases of 5% or over in four of the 10 years between 1980/81 and 1988/89. Any Government which is committing resources of this order has a clear duty to ensure that it is obtaining value for money, particularly when, as had always been recognised, it must expect in the future to meet legitimate further real terms increases in the drugs bill as a result of factors such as the projected increase in the proportion of the elderly with their markedly higher drug needs and the new treatments coming on stream not least for conditions previously untreatable.

Much progress had of course been made in pioneering more cost-effective prescribing, by which I mean the making of prescribing choices fully informed by the relativities of cost and quality of outcome for the patient. In particular the introduction of PACT in 1988, with close co-operation from the profession, represented a major step forward in making all general practitioners aware of their own prescribing patterns and costs and how they compared with those of their peers. Interestingly since the introduction of PACT there has been a significant slowing down in the rate of increase in the drugs bill which is generally considered to be at least largely due to its introduction. The object of the Indicative Prescribing Scheme is not to supplant PACT but to build on it and in particular remedy the deficiencies in relying purely on the voluntary use of PACT. Those deficiencies are essentially twofold. Firstly, all experience of voluntary prescribing initiatives shows that – very understandably – they lose their impact over time once the novelty of their introduction wears off. Secondly, it is clear that there has not been a universally positive response to PACT and it seems right that the progress stemming from PACT should not be a process from which it is open to practices, for whatever reason, to opt out.

Finally, whilst considering the position on prescribing prior to the introduction of the Indicative Prescribing Scheme, I should pay tribute to the sterling and pioneering work undertaken by officers of the Regional Medical Service (RMS). Equally, we have to recognise that the RMS suffered from external constraints on what they could achieve. Firstly, they had a relatively small number of officers (less than 50 for England as a whole) and were also undertaking a significant number of important duties unrelated to prescribing (only 10% of their overall time related to prescribing). Secondly, with their limited resources all RMS officers were asked to concentrate on liaison with relatively high spending practices. Whilst their visits to such practices showed conclusively the extent to which financial savings could be made in prescribing without in any way impairing the quality of treatment offered to patients, it did mean that RMS officers were unable to act as sources of information and advice to general practitioners as a whole and also that they were not able to influence practitioners whose prescribing could actually have been increased to serve better the interests of their patients – for instance, by making more use of new drug therapies.

The Operation of the Indicative Prescribing Scheme

Although there is a popular myth that the Indicative Prescribing Scheme is just about saving money on prescribing and not about enhancing quality, I shall nevertheless begin this Section with a discussion of the financial regime before turning to the wholly related quality initiatives.

Indicative Amounts

From 1 April 1991, each practice received an indicative amount for its drug spending from its FHSA. This is simply the best estimate that can be made of the practice's likely needs, given its historic pattern of spending, the special characteristics and interests of the practice and anticipated changes in legitimate demand for drugs. The practice then receives a monthly statement of its expenditure with an end year projection on the basis that the incidence of its spending will follow the same pattern as the previous year.

It is important to understand what indicative amounts are and what they are not. They *are* financial benchmarks against which practices' spending can be monitored and justification sought by the FHSA for marked divergencies where the reasons for this are not apparent. They are *not* financial ceilings on practices' expenditure. Indeed the Government specifically gave practices a statutory right to exceed their indicative amounts in Section 18(4) of the NHS and Community Care Act 1990 which is couched in the following terms:

> 'The members of a practice shall seek to secure that, except with the consent of the relevant Family Health Services Authority *or for good cause* [my underlining], the orders for pharmaceutical services given by them or on their behalf are such that the basic price of the services supplied pursuant to those orders in any financial year does not exceed the indicative amount notified to the practice.'

In other words practices should aim to keep to their indicative amounts unless the legitimate needs of their patients require them to be exceeded, in which case practices are free to do so.

Before leaving the subject of finance, I should add some comments on the overall financing of the FHS drugs bill. The Government has always in this area made estimates of the amount of money likely to be required in future years and has then paid out precisely the amount which is actually spent, whether or not it corresponded to the estimate made previously. Technically this is known as financing through a 'demand led non-cash limited Vote'. The introduction of the Indicative Prescribing Scheme does not alter this system; the Government will continue to meet the bill in full for the total of FHS drug expenditure which is actually incurred. For the first time we are, however, giving Regional Health Authorities (RHAs) a financial benchmark known as the 'firm budget' against which we can monitor their spending on FHS drugs and seek explanations when there are marked divergencies from the expected outcome. RHAs will very properly use the same procedure with their Family Health Services Authorities (FHSAs). This makes for sensible management accountability within the NHS for the monies we spend on FHS drugs but the important and overriding point is that it in no way interferes with Government's commitment to meet in full the FHS drugs bill.

Quality Initiatives

As already explained the Government is interested in promoting cost-effective *not* cheap prescribing. The profession itself, as again already acknowledged, has always been concerned to continue to promote quality initiatives. The Government sees its role as complementing these and in particular in ensuring the maximum dissemination of information and good practice. This is of course not a new role, as evidenced by the introduction of PACT and the provision free of charge to all general practitioners of the *British National Formulary*, the *Drug and Therapeutics Bulletin* and *Prescribers' Journal*. The Government has, however, made a further commitment by establishing two new units, the Medicines Resource Centre (MeReC) staffed by information pharmacists and the Prescribing Research Unit (PRU) under the leadership of Professor Conrad Harris. General practitioners will already be familiar with the monthly MeReC bulletin which provide advice and information on a range of drug therapies whilst the PRU is looking at the whole range of factors which influence prescribing on a longer-term basis. Two subsequent chapters in this book refer to the provision of information to doctors by the Director of MeReC, and to the use of PACT data by Professor Harris.

Another major innovation has been the appointment by all FHSAs of medical advisers on prescribing. They are obviously 'in the lead' within the FHSA on the operation of the indicative prescribing scheme and, often with pharmacist colleagues, are available to assist practices both with queries over the operation of the scheme and with other prescribing enquiries. The new system is designed to retain the achievements of the Regional Medical Service (see above), whilst removing many of the constraints under which the RMS worked. In particular, there will be more time available to the new advisers, there will be far more of them, they will be available to all practices and they will be looking at under-prescribing as well as over-prescribing. The new medical advisers have a range of backgrounds, but all have experience of general practice and many have taken up these appointments after long careers as general practitioners. They are supported in their new role by an advisory centre based alongside MeReC under the directorship of Dr Gordon England, who describes the work of this centre in a later chapter. A major task of the medical advisers will be to keep lines of communication open on all prescribing matters with their local GPs. As the medical advisers themselves would be the first to say, it is crucial that this communication should be two-way so that NHS management at all levels should be aware of the views and concerns of those who are actually prescribing to patients.

Incentive Schemes

The Indicative Prescribing Scheme includes, as was requested in principle by several local medical committees, the option of an incentive scheme for general practitioners. This is available to those who wish to group together and aim at a target below the level of their indicative amounts. If the target is reached, 50% of the target is available to be spent locally on primary care projects as jointly agreed between the relevant FHSA and general practitioners. In 1991/92 there are 16 such schemes in operation with a possible total saving of over £2m. It must be stressed that these schemes are purely voluntary and no practice is under any obligation to participate.

Sanctions

A sanctions procedure has always been available where general practitioners were believed to be prescribing excessively. The Indicative Prescribing

Scheme provides an updated procedure designed to ensure that the legitimate interests of general practitioners, as well as of the taxpayer, are fully protected. Briefly the procedure provides for an independent hearing by three qualified medical practitioners whose finding as to whether or not excessive prescribing has taken place is binding on the FHSA. If there is such a finding, there can be a financial withholding normally equivalent to the cost of the drugs excessively prescribed. There will be rights of appeal against both finding and level of withholding. There are two points to stress. Firstly, the procedure is intended as one of last resort which it is expected will very rarely have to be used. Secondly, exceeding the indicative amount does not in itself constitute proof of excessive prescribing, although it may well lead to an investigation where the reasons for the higher level than forecast of prescribing are not considered to be justifiable.

What Will the Scheme Achieve?

The intention is that the scheme should provide us with a better guarantee than that we have previously had of cost-effective prescribing, that it will provide an accountability mechanism for the very large sums of money that are spent on FHS prescribing and that it will encourage a pharmaceutical market environment where price is more closely related to efficacy and quality than has always been the case in the past.

The scheme will provide a spur to general practitioners to be more conscious of the cost of drugs and to use higher cost alternatives only where there is a roughly commensurate quality of care advantage to the patient. It will also provide a spur to cut out unnecessary prescribing completely. The much more informed monitoring of drug prescribing and expenditure that, we shall be able to undertake, will provide all levels of NHS management with better information on how FHS drug expenditure is being spent. We shall have a professional judgment as to trends in legitimate increase in expenditure as well as on areas where there may still be cause for concern that money is being wasted. Professional accountability by general practitioners for the drug spending they initiate is clearly right in principle and is perhaps less daunting than it may appear, when one realises that general practitioners are being asked to do no more than provide information on which one would have expected them to have formed their original prescribing decisions. Finally, to make pricing more sensitive to relative value and efficacy in terms of quality of care is an essential ingredient in encouraging the development of those truly innovative products which provide a significant additional benefit to patients.

Conclusions

This Chapter has been written by a civil servant and no doubt bears the hallmarks of the approach of the budding mandarin. For precisely that reason I should like to conclude by making clear that the Indicative Prescribing Scheme is not intended to be the plaything of civil servants nor indeed of NHS managers. It surely behoves all of us to remember that prescribing in the Family Health Service is an area where, as Mr Clarke readily acknowledged, we have been able to achieve a great deal for patients in recent years through the care of general practitioners. As Mrs Virginia Bottomley MP, the Minister for Health, said in a speech on 3 April 1991 talking of the role of the initiatives under the Indicative Prescribing Scheme:

'I should like to make it quite clear that it is in no way our intention to weaken the role of the general practitioner as the person who determines the drugs to be prescribed to his patient. Quite the contrary. Our aim is to provide GPs with better information on both the quality and relative cost of the medicines available so that the GP can then make the decision on whether or not to prescribe and if so what, taking full account of his personal experience and knowledge of the individual patient.'

3 Information to Doctors about Medicines

Nicholas Hough

The working paper *Improving Prescribing* stated that the indicative prescribing scheme 'will provide general medical practitioners with additional motivation, and the information and educational support, to examine critically their prescribing patterns and costs and to discuss with their medical peers ways of improving their prescribing'. In committing itself to improving the quality of prescribing in general practice, the Government stated that it would continue to pay for the distribution within the NHS of the *British National Formulary, Prescribers' Journal* and the *Drug and Therapeutics Bulletin*. Furthermore, it was announced that a centrally funded national Medicines Resource Centre had been established in Mersey Regional Health Authority to provide professional advice and information on medicinal products and matters relating to prescribing practice to all general practitioners (GPs) in England, by means of a monthly drug information bulletin.

Information on medicines is available to prescribers from a variety of other sources apart from those which are paid for by the Department of Health (DOH). These include numerous professional and commercial journals or magazines which specialise in therapeutics and prescribing, such as the *Monthly Index of Medical Specialties* (MIMS), as well as substantial amounts of literature produced by the pharmaceutical industry. In addition, there is the NHS-based National Drug Information Network, the role of which will be dealt with in more detail below.

This chapter, however, will concentrate primarily on the sources of information on medicines which are paid for on behalf of GPs in England by the DOH, with emphasis on the most recently established of these, namely the Medicines Resource Centre, or MeReC as it is also known.

The Drug and Therapeutics Bulletin

The *Drug and Therapeutics Bulletin* (DTB) is commissioned and researched by the Association for Consumer Research and published on a fortnightly basis by Consumers' Association. The DOH pays a bulk subscription on behalf of all doctors and final year medical students in the NHS in England. The DTB is independent of the DOH which has no influence on editorial policy.

Because the DTB is produced for the benefit of doctors in both hospital and general practice, it covers a very broad scope of subjects. These include, for example, new product reviews, updates on the treatment of specific diseases or medical conditions, and advice on prescribing related subjects such as the development of a practice formulary and economic prescribing. The role of allied health care professions is also examined from time to time, and in keeping with its broader viewpoint, articles on surgical procedures and other specialist topics more relevant to hospital practice are often featured. It is noteworthy that in response to *Improving Prescribing* the DTB has begun to

13

publish short notes on new drugs soon after they have been launched, without precluding a more detailed review later.

Articles appearing in the DTB are always unsigned. The reason for this is that following the writing of a first draft by an expert in the relevant field, comments are incorporated from as many as 30 to 40 other people, including outside specialists, general practitioners and members of the pharmaceutical industry. The comments of its own Editorial Panel and Advisory Council are also considered, so that the DTB, in its own words, aims to present a consensus view.

The DTB is well known for its generally forthright editorial style. Although its approach is not always appreciated by some, it has earned a great deal of respect from many doctors and pharmacists. This seems very much to be the case amongst GPs – the prescribers most frequently targeted by the marketing and sales departments of pharmaceutical companies. For many years the DTB has been the GPs only regular independent source of information on medicines.

The DTB is fairly simple in format, containing just four sides of printed text. Most issues contain two or three articles, but on occasions all four pages may be devoted to more extensive coverage of one particular subject area. The text is usually succinct, but all sources quoted are fully referenced.

Prescribers' Journal

Prescribers' Journal (PJ) is another independently produced source of prescribing information paid for on behalf of all doctors in the NHS by the DOH. There are usually about six issues per year. PJ is compiled by a representative Committee of Management supported by an Advisory Panel of experts and clinical pharmacologists. Articles are authored by specialists in the relevant field and undergo a careful review process.

The types of subjects covered mainly include the treatment and management of particular diseases or conditions, reviews of therapeutic drug groups and more general topics such as adverse drug reactions and interactions. From time to time the whole of one issue may be devoted to a series of articles presented as a symposium, for example Paediatric Emergencies. Individual articles are generally more detailed and much longer than those which appear in the DTB, and consequently each issue of PJ may contain 40 to 50 pages, although the page size is slightly smaller than A5. This means that PJ is probably used in a different way to the DTB; whereas the latter can usually be read in a matter of minutes, PJ requires the reader to spend a little more time to absorb the information and advice that it contains.

The British National Formulary

The British National Formulary (BNF) is probably the most useful and, next to *MIMS*, the most widely used primary reference source for information on medicines and prescribing. Most people will be familiar with its present distinctive format which was first introduced in February 1981. The BNF is produced jointly by the British Medical Association and The Royal Pharmaceutical Society of Great Britain. It is revised and re-published twice yearly, and is intended to be a pocket book for rapid reference.

Entries on individual drugs are organised under pharmacological or thera-peutic group headings within well structured chapters which also contain rel-evant notes to help in the choice of appropriate treatment. For each drug listed in the BNF there are short notes on indications, precautions, contra-indica-tions, side-effects and dose, as well as a list of all those pharmaceutical prepa-rations which include that drug as a main ingredient.

The BNF also provides other important information such as general guid-ance on prescription writing, prescribing for special patient groups such as children and the elderly, and prescribing in terminal care. The emergency treatment of poisoning is dealt with specifically in some detail, and there are also useful tables containing advice on prescribing in liver disease and renal impairment, prescribing in pregnancy, drugs and breast feeding, and brief notes on drug interactions.

The Joint Formulary Committee of the BNF consists of members drawn from the medical and pharmaceutical professions. A wider group of outside specialists are consulted in the preparation of each chapter, and official state-ments such as those issued by the Committee on Safety of Medicines are high-lighted in the appropriate sections. The BNF is supplied by the DOH free of charge to all doctors and pharmacists employed in the NHS. Chapter 13 describes the BNF in detail.

The BNF is an excellent source of information on medicines, and is rightly highly regarded by most prescribers as such. Together with the *Data Sheet Compendium* published by the ABPI, these two books are the main reference sources which should be readily available to all doctors and pharmacists.

The Medicines Resource Centre

The most recently established source of independent published information on medicines which is available to GPs in England is the Medicines Resource Centre, or MeReC as it is also known. MeReC came into being with the pub-lication of *Improving Prescribing* and its remit, which is defined in the working paper, is to provide professional advice and information on medicinal products and matters relating to prescribing practice to all GPs in England, with emphasis on encouraging rational, safe and cost-effective prescribing.

MeReC does this by publishing and distributing, free of charge, a monthly drug information bulletin. In addition, a series of briefings covering various therapeutic topics is also produced for FHSA medical advisers in order to facilitate their discussions on prescribing issues with GPs. MeReC is centrally funded and therefore exists within the NHS family, although it functions inde-pendently of the DOH and has complete editorial discretion with regard to the choice of subjects and content of articles which are published.

MeReC is located within Mersey Regional Health Authority. This is because over the last fourteen years the Mersey Region Drug Information Service has produced a local *Drug Information Letter*. This has been well received by doctors and pharmacists as a valuable educational aid. MeReC is therefore well placed to draw from and build on this experience.

The centre is staffed by three drug information pharmacists and a secretary, and has the guidance and support of a steering group composed equally of advisers from the disciplines of medicine and pharmacy. MeReC also liaises with the National Drug Information Network which assists in providing feedback review of draft material. It is important to point out that MeReC does not answer individual patient related drug information enquiries, which should continue to be handled by the local district or regional drug information centres. MeReC does, however, respond to any comments or questions pertaining to any advice which appears in its publications.

MeReC *Bulletins and Briefings* are prepared in-house using the latest Desktop Publishing technology. Draft articles are mostly written by MeReC staff and are circulated to a number of advisers and expert clinicians for comments and review, to ensure that the advice and information given is both accurate and practical. The bulletin layout has been designed to be easily read, and to be versatile with regard to the inclusion of tables and summary panels. Like the DTB, the *MeReC Bulletin* consists of 4 pages of A4, although the text is arranged somewhat differently. The bulletin is also printed using two colours in order to give it a slightly more attractive appearance, and to enable emphasis to be placed on important information by the use of tinted panels and highlights.

MeReC has been established only relatively recently compared with the other sources of information so far discussed, and so to some extent the centre is still developing. It is relevant in this respect to point out that MeReC became operational and started publishing its *Bulletins and Briefings*, prior to the setting of indicative amounts for GPs and before the majority of FHSA medical advisers had been appointed. Now that indicative amounts have been set and medical advisers are in post, it is to be expected that MeReC will look carefully at how the indicative prescribing scheme is progressing and consider how it should act accordingly. One area that MeReC will be examining more closely, for example, is whether the information needs of fund-holding practices differ from those of non-fundholders.

One of the main features that distinguishes MeReC from the other sources of published information described earlier, is its relationship to the other initiatives that have been introduced as a result of *Improving Prescribing*. The most significant of these is MASC, the national Medical Advisers Support Centre, and of course, the network of medical advisers themselves. MeReC is thus in a unique position to receive feedback from the prescribing 'coalface', and as a result can be reactive to any issues which require timely comment. Being co-located with MASC in Mersey RHA means that these two centres can co-ordinate their activities in order that they may respond to the drug information needs of both GPs and FHSA medical advisers.

Due to both the large number of medicines that are available on the UK market and the wide range of conditions with which patients present in general practice, MeReC's primary objective has to be to focus on those therapeutic areas where most prescribing takes place. MeReC's publications will therefore concentrate mainly on those drugs which are most frequently used by GPs in everyday practice, and not those therapeutic agents which are more the province of the hospital practitioner. It is MeReC's aim to provide clear advice on the appropriate choice of drug within the relevant therapeutic category.

According to feedback and suggestions already received from GPs and FHSA medical advisers, one of the most useful and important functions that MeReC can fulfil is to provide information on new drugs as soon as possible after they come onto the market. However, to cover every new product would be a full-time task in itself and somewhat limiting on MeReC's resources. Furthermore, there are many areas of prescribing involving more established drugs where useful advice and information can be provided. As a result, MeReC's current practice is to be selective in identifying those new products which should be reviewed as soon as it is reasonably possible to do so. New developments in the major therapeutic areas such as cardiovascular disease, asthma, infections, the central nervous system, and musculoskeletal and joint disease will be addressed as a priority.

So far the broad approach that MeReC has adopted is such that articles usually fit into one of the following categories (although these are not necessarily mutually exclusive, and there is some overlap between them):

1. new product reviews;
2. advisory/directive articles;
3. educational/informative articles;
4. matters relating to prescribing practice, and
5. miscellaneous.

MeReC's approach to new product reviews has already been discussed briefly. However, it is important to underline the fact that unless a new drug (that is to the UK market) has already gained extensive clinical experience in other countries, it may be difficult to be conclusive about its precise place in therapy at the outset. In some instances it is useful to comment on how the product is being promoted, how it is being compared with established alternative treatments, and also to respond to any premature misplaced enthusiasm either in favour or against the use of the drug.

Advisory/directive articles are intended to contain specific guidelines upon which prescribing decisions can be based. For many GPs a direct style which addresses the essential facts is exactly what is needed. This is because they may be too busy, not sufficiently interested, or not pharmacologically expert enough to review all the relevant evidence about a particular subject for themselves. MeReC has tried to adopt this approach whilst still allowing prescribers to modify the recommendations given in view of their own clinical experience. In contrast, educational/informative articles may not contain such an obvious take home message, but will present information about a group of new drugs or an update on some aspect of therapy, which may be built on in future advisory/directive articles.

Besides the medicines themselves, there are many other aspects of prescribing about which MeReC will provide information. Under matters relating to prescribing practice, the sort of topics to be included might be, for example, the advantages and disadvantages of computer generated prescribing, legislation affecting prescribing, and adverse drug reactions and interactions.

The setting of indicative prescribing amounts for GPs, and the availability of PACT data, has more than ever before focused attention on NHS drug costs. MeReC's policy with regard to the economics of prescribing is that good medicine, or in this case good prescribing, takes care of its own costs. In this respect emphasis is not placed on cost alone, but also on clinical efficacy, tolerability (safety, toxicity etc.) and the appropriateness of prescribing. Costs are always mentioned even if it is only in the form of a table of price comparisons.

In relation to this, feedback that MeReC has received suggests that those GPs who can remember them found that the 'old' cost-comparison bar-charts, which used to be produced by the DOH, were very useful in illustrating the relative prices of different drugs. Conscious of the fact that the costs of medicines should not necessarily be seen in isolation, and at the same time wanting to provide what the readership wants, MeReC has adopted the use of bar-charts, in a number of recent bulletins, following the discussion on all the other relevant clinical factors.

Future developments likely to take place in MeReC publications are the greater use of algorithms and diagrams in order to make the salient points much more succinctly, and exploring other ways of ensuring that the main points of any article are made as clearly and as simply as possible.

The Drug Information Service

In England there is a well developed NHS-based network of drug information centres which can provide the medical practitioner with information on any aspect of drug therapy. Each of the 14 English regional health authorities has a regional drug information centre and these centres co-ordinate the services provided by local and district centres, of which there are approximately 200 now in existence.

Drug information centres provide an enquiry answering service to members of all the health care professions in both hospital and community practice. Information is provided on:

(a) indication and choice of therapy, and any contra-indications;

(b) adverse effects;

(c) drugs in pregnancy and lactation;

(d) drug interactions;

(e) administration and dosage;

(f) availability, supply and costs of medicines;

(g) pharmacology and pharmacodynamics;

(h) formulation, and

(i) identification for example, foreign medicines, loose tablets, etc.

Drug information centres also produce a variety of newsletters and current awareness bulletins to meet the needs of doctors and other National Health Service staff. Several regional centres produce bulletins specifically for GPs, and, as mentioned previously, the experience of Mersey Region Drug Information Service in producing its *Drug Information Letter* was recognised in MeReC's establishment. *The Drug Information Letter* is still produced and cir-culated to doctors and pharmacists within Mersey Region, and it is important to recognise that, alongside MeReC, a number of other drug information cen-tres are also active in this way.

Locally produced bulletins and newsletters are able to address issues and problems which are peculiar to that particular geographical area. This might include, for example, prescribing at the GP-hospital interface, or prescribing for special groups of patients who might comprise a larger proportion of the local population than is the case in other parts of the country. PACT data may also highlight issues which require collaboration between the drug information centre and the FHSA's medical and pharmaceutical advisers.

Staff within the drug information network have access to a wide range of sources including textbooks, journals and computer databases either locally or via their regional centre. In addition, some centres have established specialist information and advisory services. These include:

(a) drugs in breast milk;
(b) drugs in pregnancy;
(c) drugs in dentistry;
(d) alternative medicine;
(e) drugs in renal failure;
(f) toxicology and poisoning;
(g) drugs in liver failure, and
(h) drugs in AIDS.

Requests to utilise these services can be made to the local centre; the telephone numbers of all the regional centres are listed in the BNF. From time to time a reminder to GPs about the availability of the drug information service is included in the *MeReC Bulletin*, and the drug information network is able to feedback comments and suggestions to MeReC. In a number of centres specialist primary care liaison posts have been created in recognition of the valuable role that drug information pharmacists can play in the provision of information on medicines to general practitioners.

Editor's Note: Sources of Medical Information

The chapter by Nicholas Hough on information available to doctors about medicines mentions in passing the activities of the pharmaceutical industry in this regard; these are significant and, I believe, can be valuable. Firstly, the ABPI distributes the Data Sheet Compendium free of charge to all hospitals, pharmacies, and general practitioners throughout the United Kingdom. It covers virtually all the branded medicines available on prescription in the UK, and it must be remembered that the data sheets it includes all have to be compatible with the product licences for the products to which they refer. They thus assume the status of being statutorily approved.

Secondly, advertising by pharmaceutical companies draws doctors' attention to the existence of certain products; it has to be fair, balanced and accurate, and must not mislead by implication. If it falls down on any of these issues, and, indeed, many others, it should be referred to the Code of Practice Committee, operated by the ABPI. Advertisements are also required to conform to the Advertising Regulations of the Medicines Act.

The other information activity of the industry is the phalanx of company representatives. They are expected, trained and indeed required to provide critical analyses of the products they are detailing; they also provide access to a large database of further information, maintained by the research-based companies by whom they are employed.

4 Making the Most of PACT

Conrad Harris

It has become fashionable to say that PACT (Prescribing Analysis and Cost) provides no answers, only questions, and, like most epigrams, this makes a good point at the expense of accuracy. It would be fairer, if less terse, to say that the answers PACT gives you initially can make you ask yourself questions and, when you are dealing with these, you will find some of the answers you need in PACT. To make the most of PACT you have to take into account that, as conversationalists, the three levels are very different.

Level 1

Level 1 is an extravert and not very polite. No sooner have you helped it off with its coat than it starts shouting about how you compare with other practices in your numbers of items and costs. Such bad manners are probably a cloak for its feelings of guilt; it knows that you are curious about the comparisons, but it must be well aware that no-one with any sense believes them to be important.

Why should your figures be like the local or national averages? Isn't your practice unique in all sorts of ways? Who says that being average is good? Level 1 has nothing to say to these very reasonable rejoinders; you have to answer them yourself, and the only help it offers is a slip that enables you to request Level 2 and Level 3 reports.

This rude behaviour is most likely to provoke you if you are being told that your prescribing is unaverage, but the rejoinders are just as valid if it is average. It isn't making the most of PACT to smile complacently at your averageness as you put the report away in its box: it's using the data as an anaesthetic. This is intelligent behaviour only if you plan to retire within the next three months.

Level 1's final attempt to rattle you is to hiss your percentage generic prescribing at you. This probably doesn't mean much either, since the figure combines true generic prescribing with the use of approved names for proprietary-only drugs, but it may be of interest if your main concern is to find an easy way of reducing your costs. This has nothing to do with your standard of prescribing, but there is the side-effect of saving some money for the NHS. If all GPs in England always prescribed just three drugs generically (allopurinol, ibuprofen and naproxen), this would currently save £16m a year; three more (amoxycillin, co-trimoxazole and co-amilozide) would save a further £8m.

In its own crude way, Level 1 can be quite effective in starting a conversation.

Level 2

Level 2 is narrow-minded and obsessive. It tends to mumble so much that it can be difficult to understand: probably it is ashamed of being so openly manipulative. You have to be very tolerant, or a little frightened, to have a conversation with it, because it won't talk about anything but money.

Its way of dealing with each BNF chapter takes a little getting used to, but once you have mastered the meaning of what is in the boxes, the information about your five leading cost sub-sections, drugs and preparations has its uses. Expensive hospital-shifted prescriptions will be pin-pointed, ready for you to point out to your medical adviser; and you will see where and how your highest costs were incurred. You may have been a little undiscriminating in your use of cefuroxime, or giving everyone generous supplies of paracetamol; the report will tell you.

The first of the brief tables for each chapter, headed 'Total number of items and costs by section', lifts a different veil. It gives you figures at a drug level that is pretty condition-specific, and compares them with the FHSA average. This is done nowhere else in any of the other PACT reports.

Comparative figures always attract attention, even when they don't mean much, and they are therefore likely to set you thinking. There is a good illustration of this in the Level 2 report reproduced at the end of the *The Analysis of Prescribing in General Practice*. Under Cardiovascular System the practice can be seen to be prescribing consistently fewer of all the kinds of drug used in hypertension than the area average. Is this statistically significant? Does the practice have less than the average number of hypertensive patients because of the age-structure or ethnic mix of its patients? Are its criteria for drug treatment more stringent? Is it looking hard enough for people with high blood pressure?

The answers to these queries will not be found in PACT, but PACT posed the original question without much prompting. Perhaps there ought to be more comparisons at this level of specificity, not just at overall or chapter level.

Level 3

Level 3 is a great passive creature that doesn't speak until it is spoken to. It hasn't any points it is burning to make, and leaves the content of the conversation entirely to you.

It may be easier to cope with this if you request an analysis for one chapter only – a full report can be more than 100 pages long, and this may be a conversation-stopper for anyone but the most earnest seeker after truth. You can recognise what you want more easily in a smaller picture, and usually it will be in one of three areas.

1. *Matters directly related to prescribing*

   You want:

   – to be more rational in your choice of drugs;
   – to reduce your costs;
   – to define areas in which a practice policy would be desirable;
   – to check how well you are keeping to a practice policy;
   – to create a practice formulary, working from existing preferences ;
   – to check how well you are keeping to a formulary.

   All of these represent the first or second phase of a prescribing audit, and, with all bar the first, it is pretty clear what you need to look for in your

PACT. The aim of being more rational in your choice of drugs is too vague to be useful, and to define it more closely you may have to put in some revision of your clinical pharmacology. One result of this will be to make you look askance at how often you and your partners use a host of different preparations for the same purpose.

You may be surprised, for example, to find that 20 different diuretics are being regularly prescribed: thiazides, loop diuretics, diuretics with potassium and diuretics with potassium sparers – with many examples of each kind. Why?

Basic drugs like bendrofluazide and frusemide are effective and cheap, while many of the alternatives are effective and dear. Are you clear about the clinical indications for combinations with triamterine or amiloride? If not, go and find out. Your patients may be taking them quite unnecessarily.

By the time you have assembled all the facts, you wouldn't be human if you didn't want to tell them to your partners. A new practice policy may be born.

2. *Assessing your detection of diseases*

The number of items you prescribe of some disease-specific drugs may give you a rough idea of the number of patients you are treating for those diseases. National prevalence rates should tell you how well you are doing in detecting them, but there may be local factors that make these misleading. It could be better to compare your PACT figures with those of nearby practices, especially if any of them has an interest in the condition under consideration.

3. *Teaching*

A trainee who always uses his or her trainer's FP10s and endorses them appropriately will receive a separate Trainee Level 3 report if the trainer asks for a personal Level 3. This not only yields information about the trainee's prescribing habits in a direct way, but may also be useful for teaching if it is compared with the trainer's report. A practice-aggregate report requested at the same time will show differences between the trainee's prescribing and the total practice prescribing and provide a more valid base for comparisons. Before you draw any conclusions from the differences though, it is necessary to find out if the trainee's case-mix is different from that of the principals.

Trainees will usually be involved when the partners discuss prescribing matters, and may either be interested in following up the effects of whatever decisions are made, or asked to take this on as a project. They may also have ideas of their own about using PACT. Prescribing projects are convenient because the basic data arrive in the post.

The Future

PACT (and its analogues in other parts of the UK) is far ahead of anything comparable in other countries, but it can certainly be improved. The Special Reports, described in *The Analysis of Prescribing in General Practice*, that will give separate analyses for any groups of patients chosen by a practice, have been waiting for several years to be implemented. Figures showing the extent to which a particular drug is used, with local comparison, would be interesting to many practices; and so would graphs showing trends over time in various aspects of prescribing.

Some GPs would like to have electronic access to their data so that they can make analyses of their own choosing. This is not likely to be available in the near future though; the first move will be for area data to be passed to FHSAs, and programs for Medical Advisers are already being written with this in mind.

Now and in the future the most important thing to remember, when conversing with your reports, is that they can't tell you which of your prescriptions was necessary. Thinking about that is a higher priority even than making the most of PACT.

5 Use and Development of PACT

Douglas Ball

Introduction

PACT (Prescribing Analysis and Cost) has been in operation for three years. It is a prescribing information system for general practitioners which was specially designed by the Prescription Pricing Authority (PPA) in conjunction with the General Medical Services Committee of the British Medical Association, the Royal College of General Practitioners and the Department of Health. Its aim is to give every general practitioner in England reliable, regular and prompt information which will enable GPs to:

(i) review their prescribing habits and cost;

(ii) improve their service to patients;

(iii) develop and monitor prescribing policies within the practice;

(iv) compare themselves with colleagues in the same FHSA area and nationally;

(v) improve the cost-effectiveness of prescribing within the practice;

(vi) maintain control of their prescribing.

For those who may not be familiar with the PPA, it is a special Health Authority which has two main functions: it is responsible for authorising the payment to contractors for the dispensing of NHS prescriptions; and it is responsible for the production of prescribing and drug information for England.

Historically the origins of PACT can be traced back to 1976. The provision of regular prescribing information to GPs was the main reason that the PPA went through a six year computerisation programme. Prior to the introduction of computer systems the Authority used manually to produce prescribing data known as PD2 and PD8 reports, based on prescribers' signature. The manual effort involved was such that it was nine months after the prescription was dispensed before a report could be produced and therefore the service was only available to a limited number of GPs. The first computerised information system, which went live in 1986, was based on the PD2/PD8 system; the reports therefore were very detailed and only appealed to the real enthusiast or for research projects. Herriot Watt University was funded to carry out three research projects which established that the provision of regular information in a presentable manner to GPs could have a beneficial effect on prescribing habits. These projects helped in establishing the business case for PACT.

How Prescriptions Turn into PACT Reports

Dispensing contractors, once a month, submit the prescriptions they have dispensed to the appropriate PPA office; there are 11 such offices around the country. The capture of the prescription data goes through a number of stages to ensure a high level of accuracy. Each prescription form is first numbered to provide an audit trail and record its arrival. The numbers of prescription forms and items are also used as part of calculating the monthly payments to pharmacists. Approximately 20 million prescription forms are numbered each month which equates to approximately 34 million prescription items. These items are put into the computer system each month using 1400 terminals linked to 36 ROCC minis. Patient details are not captured so confidentiality is maintained. The prescription data are then transferred over the Authority's own private and secure network to its Headquarters at Newcastle Upon Tyne onto four Bull 7000/360 mainframes. Further validation takes place using on-line terminals before calculating and reconciling payments to dispensing contractors which are currently £2.4 billion per year. Prescriber and drug information is added to this data which are then transferred via a direct link to the Authority's Information Technology Centre where the information is processed on IBM and Bull mainframes to produce PACT, Indicative Statements, Prescription Cost Analysis, and a number of other Information Services. Figure 5.1 shows a diagrammatic representation of the current system.

PACT

The PACT Prescribing Reports are based on the prescriber number stamped on the FP10 prescription pad. It is therefore up to each prescriber to be responsible for the use of his/her own prescription pad or prescriber identifier. The Authority no longer tries to identify the prescriber by signature and therefore all items prescribed against a particular prescriber identifier will be recorded against that practitioner. There are problems with the clarity and correctness of the prescriber stamp which prescribers should be aware of and consciously check on a regular basis. This applies to both manual stamp prescriptions and computer produced prescriptions.

PACT is a quarterly system; the 90 FHSAs, which are the main Department of Health users of the system are split over different quarters to even out the work load service for the Regional Medical Services. Changing the sequence of FHSAs would be a significant change but the order may be changed to ensure that all FHSAs within an RHA are in the same quarter.

There are three levels of prescribing reports:

The 'Level 1' document which every GP receives automatically. This report is practice based to reflect the practice of sharing patients and, in some cases, prescription pads. This report, which summarises prescribing for the previous quarter, has been designed to enable a practice to ascertain at a glance whether its prescribing profile is higher or lower than the FHSA average. It details the total cost of all the prescriptions during that quarter, the number of prescriptions and the average cost per prescription; and there is summary information for medicines in the six most expensive BNF therapeutic groups. The back page of the 'Level 1' report provides summary information relating to the GP to whom the report is addressed. The FHSA average figure, which is the basis for deciding if a practice is high cost or not, has caused some confusion. Page 2 of the report explains that this figure is

PRESCRIPTION PRICING AUTHORITY
HIGH LEVEL SUMMARY OF COMPUTER SYSTEMS

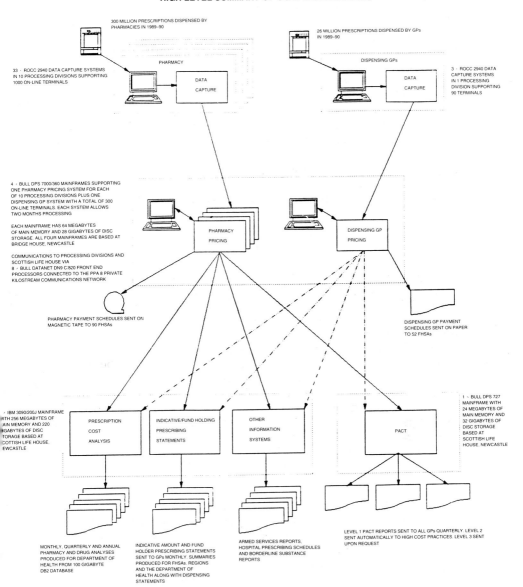

Figure 5.1

a derived figure showing what the FHSA average cost would be for a practice with the same patient list profile (see Appendix 5.1). All items personally administered are included in the PACT reports. Dispensing doctors from April 1991 now receive a combined PACT report which includes both their prescribing and dispensing patients.

A 'Level 2' report is available on request at practice or GP level. It is automatically issued to all GPs in any practice whose overall costs are 25% above the FHSA average or the practice is 75% above the FHSA average in one of the six main therapeutic groups. The 'Level 2' report highlights for the GP those areas of prescribing which it might beneficial to examine in more detail. It identifies, for each of the six major therapeutic groups, those drugs which account for the greatest portion of cost within each therapeutic group. It can identify where the use of particularly high cost medicines has affected the prescribing costs of the practice or it can be used to identify which parts of the Level 3 report to request (see Appendix 5.2).

A 'Level 3' report is available only if requested by the individual GP concerned. This report is available either at therapeutic or full catalogue level so that the GP can decide on the level of detail he or she requires. This report contains a full catalogue of the prescriptions issued and dispensed during the relevant period. The full report may be too detailed for some GPs, who may only want to concentrate on one or two therapeutic groups. To avoid GPs being swamped with detail, there is a facility to request a detailed breakdown for individual therapeutic groups. This may be a better way of utilising this report. The first three sides contain the same information as the 'Level 2' reports. The Level 3 report can be used to develop a practice formulary, as it readily identifies the common medicines prescribed by the practice. Dispensing doctors have a choice on the type of Level 3 report they require. They can request either a prescribing or dispensing or a combined report (see Appendix 5.3).

The problem in providing comparative data is that no two patient list sizes are the same and, therefore, in order to normalise those practices with a greater percentage of older patients who require a greater level of attention and hence prescriptions, the concept of prescriber units (PUs) was introduced. Patients over 65 are given a weighting factor of 3. This concept of PUs will be further refined over a period of time. If more selective information is available on patient ages and profile it may be possible to apply weightings for children and over 75s if that is shown to be the correct way to proceed.

The presentation of information in the PACT system is based on a BNF (British National Formulary) code specially designed by the PPA. This coding system has been adopted as a NHS standard for information processing and is used by a number of commercial GP system suppliers as the basis of their systems. GPs can use the reports in conjunction with the BNF to identify similar drugs which may, if used, affect their prescribing profile.

Other Aspects of PACT

A facility exists whereby a trainer can request a Level 3 report for his trainee GP. All prescriptions should have the letter 'D' clearly marked to the left of the prescriber number and the trainee should only use the same trainer's prescription pad. When a trainer requests his Level 3 report he will automatically receive a Level 3 report for his trainee. There is no facility to produce a Level 1 or Level 2 report for trainee GPs. By selective use of one prescriber pad within a practice, information can be provided on the level of repeat prescribing or on special exercises. Future developments of the service provided by the PPA will depend upon response and feed back to the GMSC and RCGP as well as to the PPA. The system is there to provide prescribing information to GPs in as meaningful and presentable manner as possible.

PACT Access by FHSAs

To enable FHSA Medical Advisers to cope with the vast amount of PACT data, FHSAs will be linked electronically to the PPA. FHSAs will be able to analyse the data in a manner which will give the Medical Adviser more time to consider the questions raised by PACT and less time handling paper. In the long term this service may eventually spread to GPs.

Appendix 5.1

PRESCRIPTION PRICING AUTHORITY INFORMATION SERVICES

Prescribing information level 1   **Quarter ended May 1991**

1. Practice Prescribing Costs

Practice	£125,757
FHSA Average	£116,942
National Average (England)	£118,867

Practice is above the FHSA Average by £8,815 or 8%
(and is above the National Average by £6,890 or 6%)

2. Practice Number of Items

Practice	£19,857
FHSA Average	£19,168
National Average (England)	£19,337

Practice is above the FHSA Average by £689 or 4%
(and is above the National Average by £520 or 3%)

3. Practice Average Cost Per Item

Practice	£6.33
FHSA Average	£6.10
National Average (England)	£6.15

Practice is above the FHSA Average by 3.8%
(and is above the National Average by 2.9%)

Appendix 5.1 (continued)

Practice Items and Total Cost by Major Therapeutic Group   Quarter ended May 1991

	Number of items	Practice is
Cardiovascular system	3,825 / 3,568	+7%
Gastro intestinal system	1,767 / 1,678	+5%
Respiratory system	1,768 / 1,621	+9%
Musculoskeletal and Joint diseases	1,432 / 1,225	+14%
Central nervous system	3,928 / 3,859	+2%
Infections	1,865 / 1,849	<1%
All other	5,272 / 5,339	−1%

EXPLANATORY NOTES

FHSA average   –   Throughout this report all the figures represented by 'FHSA Average' are based on the actual figures for the local FHSA adjusted to reflect an average practice with the same number of Prescribing Units as this practice.

National average   –   As above but based on the actual figures for England adjusted to this practice.

Prescribing unit (PU)   –   Since the proportion of elderly patients (i.e. aged 65 and over) varies between practices and the elderly receive on average three times as many prescriptions as younger patients, practice list sizes have been converted to prescribing units as follows:

No. of PUs = (No. of patients under 65) + (No. of patients 65 and over × 3)

Therapeutic groups   –   The six therapeutic groups listed are those which incurred the highest costs in England from April 1989 to March 1990, ranked in descending order of total cost. The term 'All other' includes other preparations, dressings and appliances.

Cost   –   Total Net Ingredient Cost.

Appendix 5.1 (continued)

FHSA average			Av. cost per item	
Practice is	Total cost		£	Practice is
+15%	£29,762		7.78	+6.9%
	£25,984		7.28	
+8%	£17,594		9.96	+2.7%
	£16,282		9.70	
+7%	£13,824		7.82	+1.8%
	£12,903		7.96	
+33%	£14,951		10.44	+16.4%
	£11,258		8.97	
−11%	£11,179		2.85	−12.0%
	£12,522		3.24	
+3%	£7,084		3.80	+2.4%
	£6,865		3.71	
<1%	£31,363		5.95	+2.1%
	£31,128		5.83	

EXPLANATORY NOTES

Deputising services   –   These figures represent all prescribing by Deputising Doctors who have used prescription pads stamped L and have specified the senior partner number of the practice.

Temporary residents   –   The list size shown for temporary residents is based on the same quarter of the previous year and is included in the overall list size and prescribing units figures.

Trainee doctors   –   These figures represent all prescribing by trainee doctors who have used your prescription forms having added a D in red ink to the form.

Prescribed reports   –   Where a doctor has both prescribing and dispensing patients the figures for both will be amalgamated (including list sizes).

Please refer to the PACT/IBS Technical Guide for a more detailed explanation of the above.

Appendix 5.1 (continued)

GP prescribing

Practice profile

	Prescribing list size	Patients 65 and over	Temporary residents	No PUs
	2,818	542	15	3,902
Practice	9,796	1,865	68	13,526
FHSA average	9,796	1,865	68	13,526

Practice prescribing totals

	Number of items	Total cost (£)
	4,650	33,551
Trainee doctor	0	0
Deputising services	0	0
Practice	19,857	125,757
FHSA average	19,168	116,942

Analysis by prescribing unit and patient

	Av. cost (£) per item	Items per PU	Av. cost (£) per PU	Items per patient	Av. cost (£) per patient
	7.22	—	—	—	—
Trainee doctor	0.00	—	—	—	—
Deputising services	0.00	—	—	—	—
Practice	6.33	1.5	9.30	2.0	12.84
FHSA average	6.10	1.4	8.65	2.0	11.94

Percentage of items prescribed generally

	40%
Trainee doctor	0%
Deputising services	0%
Practice	39%
FHSA average	52%
National	44%

BNF Chapter 2 Cardiovascular system

Drugs prescribed by

(Figures in brackets represent FHSA average)

Total no. of items and costs by section

		No. of items		Cost (£)	
		3,825 = 100%		£29,762.48 = 100%	
2.1	Positive inotropic drugs	194	(202)	37.11	(46.31)
2.2	Diuretics	1,122	(1,184)	3,992.63	(3,608.61)
2.3	Anti-arrhythmic drugs	14	(28)	145.29	(414.41)
2.4	Beta-adrenoceptor blocking drugs	935	(702)	8.636.37	(6,119.45)
2.5	Antihypertensive therapy	207	(306)	3.211.01	(4.761.68)
2.6	Nitrates/vasodilators/Ca-channel blockers	1,096	(846)	11,945.81	(9.521.04)
2.7	Sympathomimetics	—	(2)		(53.31)
2.8	Anticoagulants and protamine	36	(63)	27.89	(26.27)
2.9	Antiplatelet drugs	197	(193)	1,020.80	(505.58)
2.10	Fibrinolytic drugs	—		—	
2.11	Antifibrinolytic drugs & haemostatics	—	(4)	—	(44.38)
2.12	Lipid-lowering drugs	24	(39)	745.57	(883.23)
2.13	Local sclerosants	—		—	

Appendix 5.1 (continued)

BNF Chapter 2 Cardiovascular system   **Quarter ended May 1991**

Leading cost sub-section(s)	2,618 = 68%	£24,845.96 = 83%
2.2.4 Potassium sparing diuretics & compounds	513	2,784.22
2.4.0 Beta-adrenoceptor blocking drugs	935	8,636.37
2.5.5 Angiotensin-converting enzyme inhibitors	143	2,829.18
2.6.1 Nitrates	517	3,018.26
2.6.2 Calcium-channel blockers	510	7,577.93
Leading cost drugs	1,364 = 36%	£15,436.12 = 52%
2.2.4 Co-amilofruse (amiloride HCL + frusemide)	209	1,470.22
2.4.0 Atenolol	464	4,893.61
2.5.5 Enalapril maleate	91	1,896.98
2.6.1 Glyceryl trinitrate	208	1,488.19
2.6.2 Nifedipine	392	5,687.12
Leading cost preparations	732 = 19%	£8,335.15 = 28%
2.2.4 Frumil® Tab	196	1,402.66
2.4.0 Tenormin® Tab (100 mg)	172	2,090.52
2.4.0 Tenormin L.S.® Tab (50 mg)	142	1,386.60
2.6.2 Adalat Ret® Tab (20 mg)	143	2,471.66
2.6.2 Adalat Ret 10® Tab (10 mg)	78	983.71

Appendix 5.2

1. Distribution of practices in FHSA by no. items per 1000 PUs

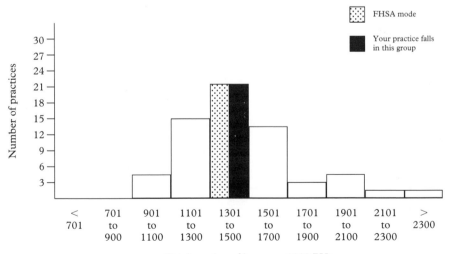

Total number of items per 1000 PUs

Appendix 5.2 (continued)

2. Distribution of practices in FHSA by total cost per 1000 PUs

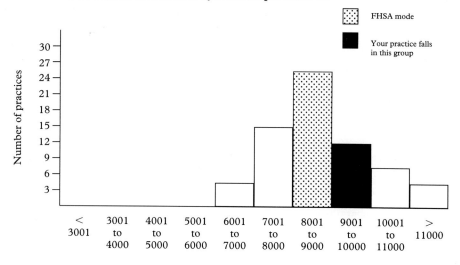

Total cost (£) per 1000 PUs

3. Distribution of practices in FHSA by average cost per item

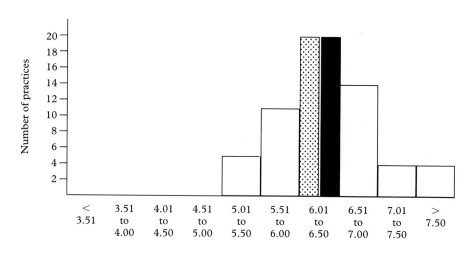

Average cost (£) per item

Appendix 5.3

		Dr. Sample	
	Quantity	No. prescriptions	Cost (£)
Promethazine hydrochloride	100	1	1.71
Phenergan® Tab 10 mg	20	1	0.51
Phenergan® Tab 25 mg	30	2	1.54
	100	1	2.55
Phenergan® Elix 5 mg/5 ml	100	7	7.00
	200	1	2.00
Terfenadine		13	15.31
Terfenadine Tab 60 mg	60	1	5.80
Triludan® Tab (60 mg)	14	3	4.05
	20	3	5.79
	24	1	2.32
	30	6	17.4
	40	11	42.57
	60	31	179.8
	100	3	29.01
Triludan® Susp 30 mg/5 ml	50	1	1.06
Triludan Forte® Tab (120 mg)	30	1	7.67
Triludan® Susp 30 mg/5 ml S/F	100	2	4.24
		63	299.71

6 Information to Patients about Medicines

Linda Stone

If any man were to ask me what I would suppose to be a perfect style of language, I would answer, that in which a man speaking to five hundred people, of all common and various capacities, idiots or lunatics excepted, should be understood by them all, and in the same sense which the speaker intended to be understood.

Daniel Defoe

The Current Situation

In the United Kingdom, other than in a few rural areas, patients requiring medication are given a prescription by their general medical practitioner. This prescription may then be presented at the community pharmacy of their choice, where the items will be dispensed. The pharmacist will place an individual label on each medicine container. This label contains dosage instructions, which are specific to that patient.

Since labels were first invented, they have been handwritten, with varying degrees of legibility. On January 1, 1984, the use of mechanically produced labels became a professional requirement. All pharmacists now produce their labels mechanically. Prior to this date, typewriters had been used in some pharmacies. Most pharmacists have since opted for computerised labelling systems, which have become increasingly sophisticated. Many incorporate patient medication records, and yet they remain simple to use. Very good use has been made of these systems, to the benefit of the patient. In addition to the obvious improvement in legibility, it is possible easily to add extra information to the label. The increasing potency of modern medicines makes this extra information critically important.

On January 1, 1987, the use of the *Guide to Cautionary and Advisory Labels for Dispensed Medicines* became a matter of professional conduct. This guide, approved by both the medical and pharmaceutical professions, has been accepted by the Joint Formulary Committee. This committee is currently chaired by Professor Charles George, and the Guide is included in the *British National Formulary* (BNF)[1] as Appendix 8. Whilst not being totally comprehensive, this guide has been a major step forward in the professional provision of patient information on a wide scale. Patients on repeat medication now receive virtually the same advice on their labels, no matter where they have their prescription dispensed. This uniformity makes the information less confusing to the patient, more acceptable to the prescriber, and is achieved very easily with modern systems.

For many patients, even such comprehensive labels are only a start. The label alone can rarely provide sufficient information. Instructions are reinforced by counselling, which has been carried out by responsible pharmacists for decades. The counselling rôle of pharmacists in hospitals and the community has been well recognised by the report of the *Independent Nuffield Foundation Inquiry into Pharmacy*,[2] Government white papers, *Promoting Better Health*,[3] and *Working for Patient Services*,[4] and by the National Health and Community Care Act.

Pharmacists in both hospital and community practice have access to a variety of high quality information sources on which to base their counselling, including *Martindale*,[5] the *BNF*,[1] *Data Sheet Compendium*,[6] the *Handbook of Pharmacy Health-Care*,[7] *Drugs in Use*,[8] and District and Regional Drug Information Units. This information is only of use because pharmacists are being given the skills necessary to enable them to communicate the wealth of relevant information which they possess. For some time, Schools of Pharmacy have been emphasising the teaching of communication skills in order to give undergraduates an appreciation of the social and behavioural sciences.[9] This is intended to give a better understanding of the context in which the information and advice will be used. Registered pharmacists also have the opportunity to acquire the same expertise through a variety of continuing education initiatives.

Another aid to patient information, which has been available for a number of years, are specific information cards. (Figure 6.1). Such cards are given out by the pharmacist at the time of dispensing. They provide an opportunity to explain some of the major problems associated with specific therapies, thus improving the patient's understanding of his, or her treatment. They are also meant to be carried at all times, so that in case of emergencies, various medical workers can be made aware of the medication being taken. At the moment, there are four cards which are available nationally: for steroids, monoamine oxidise inhibitors, lithium, and anti-coagulants.

ADVICE FOR PATIENTS ON ANTICOAGULANT TREATMENT

Always carry this card with you and show it to your doctor or dentist when obtaining treatment. Show it to your pharmacist when you are having a prescription dispensed and when purchasing medicines. As the pharmacist can advise you, it is in your own interest that you purchase all medicines from a pharmacy. Also show it to anyone giving treatment which may result in bleeding.

NAME OF YOUR ANTICOAGULANT

You should not take them unless they have been prescribed for you by the doctor who adjusts your anticoagulant dose. Aspirin may be an ingredient of other medicines, so when purchasing medicines always tell the pharmacist that you are taking an anticoagulant. Some other medicines may also interfere with the action of your anticoagulant so when you see the doctor who adjusts your anticoagulant dose always tell him about any new treatments or medicines and mention any changes, even a change of dose. If you have any doubts about your medicines ask the pharmacist or doctor.

TREATMENT

The success of your treatment depends on your taking the correct dose of anticoagu-

lant, which varies from person to person. The dose is decided by the clinic doctor after testing your blood.

BLOOD

Blood does not usually clot (coagulate) within the blood vessels. When this happens (and it may do so following illness or operation), anticoagulants are used to treat or prevent the condition by reducing the clotting power of the blood to safe levels.

FOOD AND ALCOHOL

Keep to your normal diet and do not make big changes. You may drink moderate amounts of alcohol; do not make big changes in your food and alcohol consumption.

PREGNANCY

Oral anticoagulants taken in the early weeks of pregnancy carry a small but proven risk of damaging the unborn child. If you are a

woman of childbearing years receiving oral anticoagulants, you should not embark upon a pregnancy without consulting your doctor who will be able to decide whether or not you should discontinue the anticoagulant treatment. If you find that your period is two weeks overdue and you consider that you may be pregnant while taking anticoagulants, you should make an early appointment to see your doctor.

Published by The Pharmaceutical Society of Great Britain, 1 Lambeth High Street, London SE1 7JN. Printed March 1988.

The Society acknowledges the co-operation and sponsorship of Duncan Flockhart & Co. Ltd., and Boehringer Ingelheim Hospital Division.

KEEP YOUR TABLETS IN A SAFE PLACE WELL OUT OF THE REACH OF CHILDREN

TAKING YOUR TABLETS

Remember the name and strength of the anticoagulant you are taking and always take the correct dose. Take your tablet(s) at the same time(s) each day. If necessary, use a calendar and mark off each dose by a line through the date. In this way you will be unlikely to miss a dose.

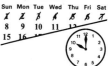

Always make sure that you have at least a week's supply of tablets in hand so that you will not run short.
NEVER miss a dose; if you do, don't take a

double dose to make up for it, but tell the clinic doctor when you next go for a blood test. If more than one dose is missed, contact your general practitioner as soon as you can for advice.

ILLNESS OR BLEEDING

In the event of illness, bleeding or apparent severe bruising, consult your general practitioner immediately. If you consult another doctor who might not know that you are having anticoagulant treatment, you must tell him, especially if an operation is necessary. Always tell your dentist.

OTHER MEDICINES

Aspirin and some other pain relieving medicines affect the clotting power of blood.

TREATMENT CARD

Carry this card with you at all times. Show it to any doctor who may treat you other than the doctor who prescribed this medicine, and to your dentist if you require dental treatment.

INSTRUCTIONS TO PATIENTS

Please read carefully

While taking this medicine and for 14 days after your treatment finishes you must observe the following simple instructions:-

1. Do not eat CHEESE, PICKLED HERRING OR BROAD BEAN PODS.
2. Do not eat or drink BOVRIL, OXO, MARMITE or ANY SIMILAR MEAT OR YEAST EXTRACT.
3. Eat only FRESH foods and avoid food that you suspect could be stale or 'going off'. This is especially important with meat, fish, poultry or offal. Avoid game.
4. Do not take any other MEDICINES (including tablets, capsules, nose drops, inhalations or suppositories) whether purchased by you or previously prescribed by your doctor, without first consulting your doctor or your pharmacist.
   NB *Treatment for coughs and colds, pain relievers, tonics and laxatives are medicines.*
5. Avoid alcoholic drinks and de-alcoholised (low alcohol) drinks.

Keep a careful note of any food or drink that disagrees with you, avoid it and tell your doctor.

Report any unusual or severe symptoms to your doctor and follow any other advice given by him.

| M.A.O.I. |

Prepared by The Pharmaceutical Society and the British Medical Association on behalf of the Health Departments of the United Kingdom.

Printed in the UK for HMSO 8217411/150M/9.89/45292
Revised Sep. 1989

I am a patient on—

STEROID
TREATMENT

which must not be stopped abruptly

and in the case of intercurrent illness may have to be increased

full details are available from the hospital or general → practitioners shown overleaf

STC1

INSTRUCTIONS

1 *DO NOT STOP taking the steroid drug except on medical advice. Always have a supply in reserve.*
2 *In case of feverish illness, accident, operation (emergency or otherwise), diarrhoea or vomiting the steroid treatment MUST be continued. Your doctor may wish you to have a LARGER DOSE or an INJECTION at such times.*
3 *If the tablets cause indigestion consult your doctor AT ONCE.*
4 *Always carry this card while receiving steroid treatment and show it to any doctor, dentist, nurse or midwife or anyone else who is giving you treatment.*
5 *After your treatment has finished you must still tell any doctor, dentist, nurse or midwife or anyone else who is giving you treatment that you have had steroid treatment.*

Printed in the UK for HMSO 4/90 8196700 388m 15474

	Name and Address	Tel No.	Treatment was commenced on........................
			DRUG	DATE	DOSE
Patient					
General Practitioner					
Hospital					
Consultant or Specialist	Hospital No.				

THINKING ABOUT STARTING A FAMILY?

Because Lithium can effect the unborn baby do NOT become pregnant without first talking to your doctor. If you are pregnant tell your doctor now.

Published by the Royal Pharmaceutical Society of Great Britain, 1 Lambeth High Street, London, SE1 7JN.
Printed April 1989.

The Society gratefully acknowledges the co-operation and sponsorship of Delandale Laboratories Ltd., Norgine Ltd., Smith Kline and French Laboratories Ltd., and Lagap Pharmaceuticals Ltd.

KEEP YOUR TABLETS IN A SAFE PLACE WELL OUT OF THE REACH OF CHILDREN.

PLEASE RECORD YOUR BLOOD LEVEL OF LITHIUM

DATE TAKEN	BLOOD LEVEL	DAILY DOSE

LITHIUM
TREATMENT CARD

CARRY THIS CARD WITH YOU AT ALL TIMES. SHOW IT TO ANY DOCTOR OR NURSE WHO TREATS YOU AND ANY PHARMACIST YOU BUY MEDICINES FROM.

NAME ....

PREPARATION OF LITHIUM ....

Should a different proprietary product be prescribed, the card must be suitably endorsed.

HOW SHOULD I TAKE THE TABLETS?

Swallow each tablet whole or broken in half, with water. Do NOT chew or crush it. Try to take the dose at the same time each day.

WHAT SHOULD I DO IF I MISS A DOSE?

Do NOT double your next dose. If you find you have missed a few doses, start taking your usual dose on the day you remember and tell your doctor.

WHY MUST I HAVE A BLOOD TEST?

This is to check the amount of lithium in your blood. It is very important to have the correct amount because too much can be dangerous. Take the blood test ABOUT 12 HOURS AFTER the last dose of lithium.

CAN I DRINK ALCOHOL?

It is safe to drink SMALL quantities.

CAN I TAKE OTHER MEDICINES WITH LITHIUM?

Some medicines can change the amount of lithium in the blood. These include diuretic (water) tablets and capsules, some pain killers and some indigestion mixtures and laxatives. So check with your doctor or pharmacist before taking other medicines.

Please note: It is safe to take aspirin and paracetamol but not ibuprofen.

WHAT ELSE ALTERS THE LITHIUM LEVEL?

The level can be altered by the amount of fluids you drink, changes in the amount of salt in your food, sweating more than usual (in hot weather, fever or infection), severe vomiting, severe diarrhoea and a low salt diet. Check with your doctor if any of these things happen.

SIGNS OF A HIGH LITHIUM LEVEL

Vomiting, severe diarrhoea, unusual drowsiness, muscle weakness and feeling very giddy may mean that your level of lithium is too high. Stop taking the tablets and talk to your doctor IMMEDIATELY.

DOES LITHIUM HAVE SIDE EFFECTS?

Some slight effects (such as sickness, shaking) may occur at first but they usually wear off if blood tests are normal. Discuss this with your doctor. Some patients may gain weight but this can be prevented with a sensible diet.

HOW LONG WILL I HAVE TO TAKE LITHIUM?

Lithium is a way of preventing illness so you may have to take it for many years. Never stop taking the tablets without asking your doctor.

Figure 6.1: Information cards: for example anticoagulants, steroids and lithium.

NOTES FOR THE PATIENT

HOW TO USE YOUR NASAL DROPS OR NASAL SPRAY

NASAL DROPS

(1)   First, gently blow your nose to clear the nostrils, then
      sit down.

(2)   Draw sufficient solution into the dropper, and tilting
      the head back, place the required number of drops
      (2 or 3 if not stated) into one or both nostrils - as
      directed.

(3)   By *carefully* tilting the head back further, the drops
      will spread gradually throughout the nasal passage.

(4)   Remain with your head in this position for about
      two minutes, breathing only through the mouth.

ILLUSTRATION OVERLEAF

NASAL SPRAY

(1)   Place the nozzle to your nostril covering the other
      nostril with the thumb of your free hand.

(2)   Spray the medicament into the nose whilst breathing
      in *very* gently to take it into the nose but no further.

(3)   Breath out through your mouth.

(4)   Repeat for other nostril.

KEEP ALL MEDICINES OUT OF THE REACH OF CHILDREN

It is inadvisable to use nasal drops or nasal spray for any
length of time, without asking your doctor.

Pharmacy Practice Group
University of Aston in Birmingham © 8094

How to use your Nasal Drops

NOTES FOR THE PATIENT

HOW TO USE YOUR EYE OINTMENT

(1)   First wash hands and then gently clean the
      eyelids.

(2)   Next, gently pull the lower lid downwards, and
      direct your gaze upwards.

(3)   *Carefully* place a thin line of ointment along
      the inside of the lower eyelid. Avoid touching
      the eyelid with the tube nozzle if possible.

ILLUSTRATION OVERLEAF

(4)   Next close your eye, and move the eyeball
      from side to side. *Gentle* massage will also
      help to spread the ointment.

Initially your vision may be blurred, but will soon
be cleared by blinking. *DO NOT RUB THE EYE AT
THIS STAGE*

Be sure to complete the course of the treatment as
directed.

Do not share the eye ointment with anyone else.

Store in a cool dark place

KEEP ALL MEDICINES OUT OF THE REACH OF
CHILDREN

Pharmacy Practice Group
University of Aston in Birmingham © 8093

How to use your Eye Ointment

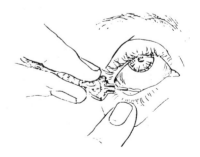

Figure 6.2:   Jepson's leaflets.

Also, workers such as Jepson,[10] have devised a variety of generic leaflets which refer to the method of use of a product, rather than to specific, individual products. (Figure 6.2). These cover various external preparations, including drops, pessaries, creams, inhalers and tablets. Although not ideal, this type of leaflet provided a useful start for the provision of written information. However, they were not used as widely as they might have been.

Patient information leaflets are now being supplied by some, but not all, manufacturers. In particular this is true with products that are normally dispensed in original packs. In order to fill the gap for those products which do not come with a leaflet, professionals are using their own initiative. Some are devising leaflets which are produced locally, and some are using computerised labelling systems which also provide a computer generated patient information leaflet.

If the information in a leaflet is intended as an aid to counselling, and a reinforcement of information already given, then it must be understood by the recipient.

At least one million adults in the United Kingdom have a reading age of less than 9 years.[11] This is certainly a significant underestimate of the situation with the numbers involved being at least two to three million, if not many more. In 1990, it was reported that 25% of 16–20 year olds admitted having difficulties with reading.[12] This means that there are nearly one million problem readers in this age group alone.

This does not take into account the problems of ethnic groups. Here, people may or may not be able to read, but where they cannot speak English, they are also unlikely to be able to read English. It has been estimated that between 25% and 35% of some immigrant communities are illiterate. Kaur and Dobrzanski studied inpatients of Indian and Pakistani origin in Bradford Royal Infirmary.[13] In their group, 71% were unable to read or write English, and more than half admitted to being unable to read their own ethnic origin language. The majority relied on their children to read the label. This places an intolerable burden on sometimes quite small children, whose understanding and reading ability is unknown. A state of affairs such as this deeply undermines the safety message that appears on every bought, and dispensed, medicine in the United Kingdom: 'Keep out of reach of children'.

Apparently, there has been no research to determine a national average reading age in this country. What is known is that an average reading age of 8½ to 9 years is consistent with the country's best selling national news-paper, the 'Sun,' which has a circulation approaching four million. The *Sun* is read by about 13 million people every day. If readers are presented with information about which they have no prior knowledge, such as a newly diagnosed health problem, then it is considered essential to prepare it for a reading age 18 months lower, i.e. 7 to 7½ years. This age is also appropriate for those children who read and translate instructions for their elders. The problem of poor reading seems unlikely to be rectified in the near future. At the end of 1990, it was reported that 20% of seven-year-olds could not make simple words and phrases.[14] This equates to over one million children still being illiterate after at least two years at school.

The Problems

The object of providing patients with more information is to improve their understanding of their medical condition and its treatment, not to confuse.

Between 37% and 54% of what doctors tell patients is forgotten when they leave the surgery.[15] Extrapolate that to the one million prescription items dispensed every day by community pharmacies in England and Wales to give an idea of the size of the problem faced by pharmacists. Counselling and labels are not enough. Patients, although more relaxed when they reach the pharmacy than in the doctor's surgery, are still liable to forget a significant proportion of what is said. Professor George has been involved in a series of studies using the 'Bloggofen' type of leaflet (Figure 6.3). This is a well compiled leaflet containing simple information on one side, with more complex information on the other. In his studies, George[16] concluded that leaflets do affect knowledge. He also found that patients who received their leaflets from a pharmacist were more knowledgeable and significantly more satisfied than were those who received the same leaflet from their General Practitioner. He was uncertain whether or not this extra knowledge affected compliance.

Linda Dodds,[17] in a study on the effects of information leaflets on compliance with antibiotic therapy, found that the additional information did result in a significant improvement in drug taking behaviour.

Good, properly designed, patient information leaflets will reinforce the information which has been given, and improve compliance, but they must be widely available.

Just as improved consistency on labels has helped, so will improved consistency in leaflets. Leaflets supplied with generic products do not all contain the same information and advice, and not all products are supplied with leaflets. In spite of proposed European legislation, the time when all products in the United Kingdom are supplied with a manufacturer's leaflet is still some way off. Until that time is reached, pharmacists will continue to exercise their professional discretion. Stocks of leaflets and warning cards are inclined to run out, or they may become lost in the post. Locally produced leaflets vary from excellent to not so good, and may not necessarily address the real problem. Computer printed leaflets are, potentially, a minefield. Several different labelling and record systems are in common use, with differing levels of sophistication and quality of data. The variations possible in the words used on a label are limited when compared to a leaflet. In addition, the very real problems of liability when product specific advice does not originate from the manufacturer cannot be ignored. Consistency of information seems to be hard to achieve.

Work done in the United States[18] showed that the approximate reading level of medicine directions on over the counter preparations was 14 to 15 years. This gives a potential reading age gap between existing labels and the just literate sections of the population of at least six years. Table 6.1 illustrates the types of words which are not understood. It is based on a questionnaire sent out to literacy and language schemes throughout Great Britain. Specifically, adult literacy and English as a Second Language students underlined the words, commonly found on medication labels, which they did not understand. The average reading age of those surveyed was found to be 9½ years.

What you should know about Bloggofen

**Please read this carefully before you start to take your medicine.
This leaflet does not contain the complete information about your
medicine. If you have any questions or are not sure about anything ask
your doctor or pharmacist.**

The name of your medicine is Bloggofen (generic name)
This is one in a group of medicines called Anti-Inflammatory
Analgesics. These can relieve pain such as headache, toothache,
arthritis and period pain.

Things to remember about Bloggofen

1 Make sure it is safe for you to take Bloggofen
(see the back of this leaflet). ◆

2 Take your medicine
**as directed by your doctor and
look at the label** on your medicine.

3 Bloggofen sometimes cause problems.
You can find these listed on the back of this leaflet. ★

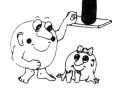

4 Keep your medicine **out of reach
of children.**

**5 Remember to return any
unused tablets** to your pharmacist or
flush them down the toilet.

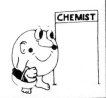

CHEMIST

You will find more about Bloggofen on the back of this leaflet.   *Reg. No:*

Figure 6.3: Bloggofen leaflet – both sides.

Bloggofen is an Anti-Inflammatory Analgesic. Anti-Inflammatory Analgesics can relieve pain such as headache, toothache, arthritis, and period pain. Doctors sometimes prescribe this medicine for other purposes; consult your doctor for information.

◆ Before taking your medicine

- Are you already taking aspirin or another drug used to treat arthritis?
- Have you had an allergic reaction or wheezing after taking aspirin?
- Have you experienced stomach discomfort, felt like being sick or had heartburn after taking aspirin?
- Have you had a stomach ulcer previously?
- Are you on medicines for thrombosis (eg Warfarin) or gout?
- Are you pregnant?
- Do you suffer from liver or kidney disease?

If the answer is YES to any of these questions tell your doctor or pharmacist.

Taking your medicine

- It is important to take your medicine at the right times. You must take it as directed by your doctor. The label will tell you how much to take and how often. If it doesn't or you are not sure, *ask your doctor or pharmacist.*
- Tablets should be swallowed with a glass of water or milk, after meals. The first dose of the day may be taken before breakfast.
- If you forget to take a dose take another as soon as you remember. Then go on as before.
- In the event of an accidental overdose contact your nearest hospital casualty department or tell your doctor immediately.

★ After taking your medicine

This medicine sometimes causes side-effects in some people.
If you get any of the following, stop taking the tablets and tell your doctor.
- Skin troubles such as rash or itching for the first time.
- Wheezing.
- You develop stomach discomfort or heartburn for the first time.
- You vomit blood or pass tarry stools.

Storing your medicine

- Keep your tablets in a safe place where children cannot reach them. Your tablets could harm them.
- If your doctor decides to stop the treatment, return any left over tablets to the pharmacist or flush them down the toilet. Only keep them if your doctor tells you to.

What's in your medicine

- Bloggofen tablets are purple in colour and come in three sizes containing either x mg, y mg, or z mg of approved name(s) of active ingredient(s).
- They contain the following preservatives or other inactive ingredients.

REMEMBER: This medicine is for YOU. Only a doctor can prescribe it for you. Never give it to others. It may harm them even if their symptoms are the same as yours.

The Product Licence for Bloggofen is held by (name and address)
The leaflet is produced in accordance with guidance issued by the Association of the British Pharmaceutical Industry. The information in it applies only to Bloggofen.

Figure 6.3: continued.

TABLE 6.1: **Understanding labels**

Words	% of ESL students who underlined difficult words $N = 144$	% of AL students who underlined difficult words $N = 392$
Symptoms	79.9	46.5
Exceed	75.8	37.1
Persist	71.8	40.6
Stated	59.7	33.9
Consulted	49.7	31.7
Otherwise	40.3	29.2
Directed	39.6	33.9
Unless	38.3	24.0
Dose	33.6	10.1
Adults	26.8	19.3

Health professionals are not alone in using words that the general public cannot understand. Table 6.2 is from a publication for Road Safety Officers, *Adult Understanding of Terms*.[19] It illustrates the scale of the problem. Table 6.3 shows the sort of 'technical words, in driving terms, that were not understood'. Many of them are everyday phrases and expressions.

Some Solutions

In assessing a number of patient specific drug information leaflets in 1987, Bailie and Bennett stated:

'Many existing leaflets were too verbose, containing too much information or written in medical jargon or inaccurate'.[20]

If a document looks confusing, then it will be confusing. Few of its prospective readers will keep reading long enough to find out to what extent they understand the words. Assuming that the words chosen are capable of being understood by the target audience, there are various ways in which a leaflet may be made more 'reader friendly' and attractive. How a document is compiled is dependant upon what is being said, and to whom, but certain factors are common to all good document design. Typeface size and style are important. Novelty typefaces should not be used. *Italics* and CAPITALS should be avoided, **bold type** is a much better way of providing emphasis. The 'x' height or size of the type is also important, but is constrained by the size of the document and the amount of information to be conveyed (Figure 6.4).[21] Open typeface is easier to read than a similar sized condensed typeface. Short, simple sentences which avoid long, complicated words are simpler to understand.

TABLE 6.2: **Percentages of 'correct' answers – given by male and female respondents**

	Male	Female	Percentage differences
Technical terms	36	28	8
Non-technical terms	44	42	2
Percentage differences	8	14	

TABLE 6.3:   Technical words – comprehension levels for terms tested

Term	All respondents Correct answer %	Percentage giving correct answers Driver %	Non-driver %
Acceleration lane	9	15	2
Alter course	39	41	35
Aquaplaning	12	21	3
Black ice	45	60	34
Blind spot	18	32	8
Box junction	37	53	27
Brake fade	4	5	4
Camber	9	14	6
Carriageway	22	32	16
Central island	54	48	59
Central refuge	23	34	14
Central reservation	12	23	5
Chevrons	4	6	2
Clearway	32	51	18
Coasting	37	68	14
Collision course	26	41	14
Convenient lane	28	35	22
Count down sign	26	56	7
Crawler lane	20	28	9
Cul de sac	72	76	69
Cutting in	35	56	20
Deceleration lane	45	69	30
Disengage	21	36	8
Diversion	57	61	55
Driver technique	30	35	28
Dual carriageway	27	38	17
Filtering	4	4	3
Filter lanes	16	25	9
Flyover	28	33	23
Full beam	63	74	54
Gradient	57	79	36
Guard rail	31	35	29
Hard shoulder	38	44	26
Hatched markings	1	2	0
Hold back (from overtaking)	19	23	13
Impaired control	18	19	20
Intersection	32	40	23
Lane discipline	48	65	15
Lane lines	1	2	0
Lock the wheels	4	7	0
Manoeuvre (to)	28	35	22
Marker post	3	4	1
Motorway interchange	25	42	11
Nearside	63	72	55
Offside	34	55	17
Pelican crossing	38	40	35
Reflective studs	51	56	47
Revving up	20	30	10
Right of way (to have)	25	25	24
Roadworthy	56	63	52
School crossing patrol	78	76	81
Self cancelling indicator	45	67	30
Separation distance	53	58	49
Single track road	21	28	10

TABLE 6.3 (continued)

Term	All respondents Correct answer %	Percentage giving correct answers Driver %	Non-driver %
Skidding	16	14	16
Slip road	23	33	14
Speed differential	10	21	2
Stalling	48	49	49
Stopping distance	15	15	13
Straddle (a white line)	46	53	39
Synchromesh	3	6	0
Tail lights	79	86	71
Three lane road	24	45	9
Traffic block	52	60	45
Traffic islands	36	40	33
Two way traffic	71	77	69
U-turn	39	56	29
Uncontrolled crossing	17	18	12
Underpass	45	50	41
Warning triangle	31	33	28
When you hold the steering wheel at ten-to-two	49	70	34
Zone of vision	40	44	35

Headings must be clearly identified so that the reader can find information quickly, without reading large sections of text. The use of 'white' space and margins are important to give a balanced appearance which is not forbidding. The colour of the print in relation to the background exerts a strong influence on the looks and readability. Strong colours on a light background have been found to be much more acceptable than light colours on a dark ground, or dark colours on a dark ground. The overall length of a leaflet is also critical; overwhelm the readers, and they will give up in despair. Illustrations may be

Leading and word spacing

The space between the bottom of the letters on one line and the top of the letters on the line below is called **leading** (pronounced 'ledding').
See Figure

Figure
Leading, type size and word spacing.

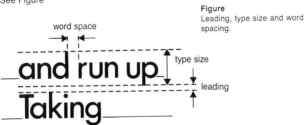

The leading should be about a quarter of the type size. If it is much less than this, the type will look cramped and crowded. If it is much more, the lines of type will look too far apart.

Figure 6.4: Diagram from 'Instructions for Consumer Products'.

FRUSEMIDE
Other name : Lasix

Why is this drug prescribed?
Frusemide acts on the kidneys causing them to eliminate excess water and salt from the body into the urine. It is used to treat high blood pressure, swelling caused by water retention, heart disease and other medical problems.

What storage conditions are necessary?
Keep this medicine in the container given. Do not be concerned if it turns dark after a while. This does not make it less effective.

When should it be used?
Frusemide is usually taken once or twice a day. Follow carefully the instructions on your prescription label. If you are taking it twice a day it is best to take one dose in the morning and one in the afternoon. If you take Frusemide late in the day or at night, it may cause you to frequent the toilet during the night.

What should I do if I forget to take a dose?
Take the missed dose as soon as you remember it but do not take two doses at one time to make up for the missed one.

How should it be used?
Your prescription label gives specific instructions regarding the dosage. It may be necessary to take this drug continuously for one to two weeks before the full effects can be realised.

What side effects can this drug cause? What can I do about them?
Weakness, muscle cramps, light headedness, ringing in the ears, dizziness. Contact your doctor.

What special instructions should I follow?
Always finish the medicine prescribed for you. It must be taken regularly to be effective. Do not forget to take your medicine and do not skip doses. Frusemide begins to work in about an hour and is effective for 4-8 hours afterwards. Therefore plan your activities accordingly to make sure you have access to a toilet in that 8-hour period. If the doctor puts you on a special diet or prescribes other medication for you while you are on Frusemide, be sure to follow instructions very carefully. Your doctor might want to monitor your response to this drug closely. Therefore keep in touch with him/her and be sure to keep all your check-up appointments. Weigh yourself daily or on alternate days. If you start to gain weight rapidly or your hands or feet start to swell, contact your doctor. Pinch the top of your hand. If the skin remains puckered after you let go, contact your doctor.

What other precautions should I follow while using this drug?
Frusemide must be taken regularly to be effective. Check your medicine before vacations or business trips to ensure ample supply.

When in doubt consult your pharmacist.

✚ National University Hospital
PHARMACY

5 Lower Kent Ridge Rd • Singapore 0511 • Tel: 772 5181, 772 5009

Printing sponsored by HOECHST (S) PTE LTD

1/8/87

Figure 6.5: Singapore leaflet.

腹安酸 FRUSEMIDE

别名：速尿

Other name : Lasix

这药的作用是什么？

腹安酸能促使肾把体内过多的水份与盐份排入尿液里。它用于治疗高血压、水肿、心脏病和其他医疗上的问题。

怎样贮藏此药？

把药保存在原来的药瓶内。药色变暗效力依然保存，不必顾虑。

什么时候用药？

通常每日服药1或2次。遵照标签上的说明服药。每日服药2次的；宜上、下午各服一剂药。傍晚或晚上服药，会造成夜尿多。

若忘了服药该怎么办？

想起时即补服，但勿加倍份量以补回漏了的一份。

怎样用药？

药物的标签上清楚说明用药的剂量。此药可能要继续服用1至2个星期后，才发挥其最大效能。

服药后会引起什么副作用？该怎么办？

衰弱无力、肌肉痉挛、轻度头痛、耳鸣和头晕，应与医生联络。

在服药期间要注意哪些预防措施？

把药服完。按时服药以期收效。勿漏服或省服。此药在服后1小时药性发作，可维持4到8小时，安排好在这8小时内方便到厕所去。医生指定特别的饮食或另处方的药均得遵守。医生亦可能要观察病人对药性的反应，故病人须与医生保持联络，并依约接受检查。病人每日或每隔1日要测量体重。倘发现体重速增或手脚浮肿，应与医生联络。把手背的皮肤拧起，松手后，若皮肤仍皱着，也应与医生联络。

在服药期间要注意什么特别事项？

必须按时服药，才能收效。因渡假或公事出远门者，须先检查药物，备足药量。如有疑问，可向药剂师请教。

When in doubt consult your pharmacist.

✚ **National University Hospital**

PHARMACY

5 Lower Kent Ridge Rd • Singapore 0511 • Tel: 772 5181,

Printing sponsored by HOECHST (S) PTE LTD

1/8/87

Figure 6.5: continued.

of help, provided that they are of a general nature. Pictogramme-type symbols are not easily understood without a comprehensive, and expensive, education campaign.

Information in leaflets must be information which communicates. Information for its own sake just creates an ineffective means of communication which frequently confuses. Leaflets must be non-promotional and easy to read. They should not be filled with quantities of information that the manufacturer believes will reduce his liability should a patient suffer any ill effects, such as the leaflets produced for oral contraceptives. The problems of minority groups who are unable to communicate in English and of English speaking people who cannot read must be addressed. This is possible. Figure 6.5 illustrates one of a series of well thought out leaflets from Singapore, which are produced in English and Chinese, the two indigent languages. Although not necessarily ideal in the light of what is known about document design, they are a very good start.

Careful design will ensure that future leaflets are not as formidable as some current examples.

It is important that progress is made in the field of patient information leaflets more rapidly than at present.

The ABPI has endorsed George's design. Nobody else has yet to suggest anything better. Complex concepts are difficult to convey simply. Simplifying words may mean that patients whose reading ages are above the national average misunderstand. The use of 'Plain English' does not provide the simple solution that professionals seek. There is no simple solution. The double sided leaflet allows information to be supplied at two different levels of understanding. The more literate, better educated patients are quite capable of seeking, and understanding, more detailed information, if they want it. Some, with a lesser ability to understand will also be able to derive benefit from such a leaflet.

Leaflets, labels and counselling must be designed to help those who are either unable to ask, or do not know how to ask, for themselves.

'Except ye utter by the tongue words easy to be understood, how shall it be known what is spoken? For ye shall speak into the air'.   (*St. Paul*).

References

1. British National Formulary (1991). Number 22. London, British Medical Association and Royal Pharmaceutical Society of Great Britain.
2. Pharmacy (1986). The Report of a Committee of Inquiry appointed by the Nuffield Foundation. London. *The Nuffield Foundation.*
3. Promoting Better Health (1987). The Government programme for improving primary health care. London, HMSO.
4. Working for Patients (1989). London, HMSO.
5. Martindale (1989). The Extra Pharmacopoeia, 29th Edition, Edited by J. E. F. Reynolds, London, *Pharmaceutical Press.*
6. ABPI Data Sheet Compendium 1990–91. London, Datapharm. 1990.
7. Handbook of Pharmacy Health-Care (1990). Diseases and Patient Advice. Edited by R. J. Harman. London, *Pharmaceutical Press.*
8. Drugs in Use (1991). Clinical case studies for pharmacists. Edited by L. J. Dodds. London, *Pharmaceutical Press.*
9. Anon. (1989). Working Party recommends social sciences teaching to undergraduates. *Pharmaceutical Journal* 243, 228.

10. Anon. (1989). Notes for the patient. *Pharmaceutical Journal* **221**, 287.
11. A language for life (1975). London, HMSO.
12. Use and literacy research press release made on May 23, 1990, by the Adult Literacy and Basic Skills Unit, London.
13. Kaur, M. and Dobrzanski, S. (1988). Pharmacy counselling for patients of Indian/Pakistan origin. *British Journal of Pharmacy Practice* **10**, 345–350.
14. Anon. (1990). Home news, *Sunday Times*, December 30, 1990.
15. Lex, P. (1979). Memory for medical information. *British Journal of Social and Clinical Psychology* **18**, 245–250.
16. Anon. (1987). Leaflets found to help patients – but who should issue them? *Pharmaceutical Journal* **238**, 700–701.
17. Dodds, L. J. (1986). Effects of information leaflets on compliance with antibiotic therapy. *Pharmaceutic Journal* **236**, 48–51.
18. Understanding labels (1980). Problems for poor readers. *Adult Literacy Support Services Fund.*
19. Adult Understanding of Terms (1982). A guide for road safety officers. *County Road Safety Officers Association.*
20. Bailie, G. R. and Bennett, S. (1987). Development of patient-specific drug information leaflets. *Pharmaceutical Journal* **238**, 803–804.
21. Instructions for consumer products (1988). London, HMSO.

7   The Economics of Prescribing and Underprescribing

George Teeling-Smith

Health expenditure is rising everywhere, as a result of advances in technology, consequent increases in life expectancy, and greater expectations of better care from the public. It is therefore becoming increasingly important to ensure that the money spent on health care is used as effectively as possible. The diagram in Figure 7.1 shows very simply the principles of health economics, which is the science concerned with the optimum use of health care resources. On the left there are the same classical 'inputs' as in any industry – manpower, materials and capital. On the right there are the 'outcomes' of medical care: these are more difficult to measure than the output of most other industries, which can be simply measured in units of production. In the centre of the diagram lies the National Health Service, which converts the inputs into outcomes. The efficiency with which it does this is also more difficult to measure than in most other industries where 'profit' is the classical measure of industrial efficiency. Profit is clearly irrelevant in the case of the National Health Service, and other proxy measures of efficiency must therefore be employed. This chapter is largely concerned with the ways in which this efficiency is measured, by relating outcomes to the resources used in terms of 'cost effectiveness'. It emphasises that the use of modern and relatively expensive medicines can be one of the most cost-effective ways of providing medical care. However, it is important to realise that this cost-effectiveness will often only be appreciated if health care costs as a whole are taken into consideration, instead of viewing pharmaceutical costs in isolation. Most often, the savings from the use of modern and relatively expensive medicines will occur in the hospital sector.

Table 7.1 shows a classic analysis in which the reduction in the use of hospital beds in Britain's National Health Service between 1957 and 1982 for nine groups of disease is compared against the cost of *all* pharmaceuticals pre-

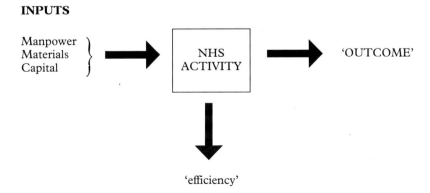

Figure 7.1:   The NHS model.

53

TABLE 7.1:   Savings from nine groups of diseases

	Bed days 1957	Beddays 1982	Hospital savings £ million
Asthma	394,331	297,281	7
Epilepsy	500,053	247,352	19
Glaucoma	148,969	89,096	4
Hypertension	1,204,277	185,510	77
Bronchitis	1,262,028	471,459	60
Skin disease	1,122,385	996,204	9
Tuberculosis	6,886,552	106,323	509
Other infections	2,766,190	553,947	167
Mental illness	52,487,000	27,324,630	847
Total saving			1,699
Manufacturers' cost of *all* pharmaceuticals			1,225
'Cost benefit pay-off'			474

scribed in the latter year.[1] Not all the reduction in hospital beds is, of course, due to better medicines; but on the other hand the cost of medicines relates to many more than just the nine groups of diseases shown. Above all, the comparison indicates the relative order of magnitude of potential hospital savings when compared to the cost of medicines.

Table 7.2 shows a specific more recent example where medicines could pay for themselves.[2] It is estimated that the use of hormone replacement therapy (HRT) could be associated with a reduction in the number of hip fractures by 50%. On this basis, the cost of the medicine saves more than twice its value in reduced surgical and hospital costs. Admittedly the savings occur at a later date than the cost of the HRT, but it is likely that the escalation of hospital costs will largely offset the effects of 'discounting' future expenditures.

A striking example of savings from the use of medicines (which is discussed again below) comes in the use of medicines to control hypertension and hence to reduce the number of strokes. It is estimated from general practice statistics that if there had been no reduction since 1954/55 the number of new strokes per 1,000 population aged 45–64 would have been 2.4 in 1981/82 instead of the actual figure of 1.75.[3]

Without a reduction of this magnitude, it is estimated that the cost of strokes to the National Health Service would have been £754 million instead of £550 million in 1985. This saving of £204 million can be viewed against the total cost of all medicines for the treatment of hypertension of £185 million. Thus the saving to the health service from strokes alone more than pays for the cost of all anti-hypertensive medication.

TABLE 7.2:   HRT and hip fracture – 1985

Hospital costs of hip fracture	£128 m
Probable saving: 50%	£ 64 m
Cost of HRT	
25% at high risk 10 years treatment	£ 31.25 m
Saving to health service	£ 32.75 m

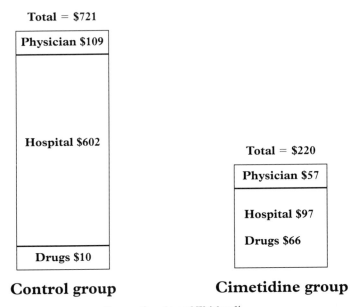

Source: Geweke and Weisbrod[4]

Figure 7.2:   Average annual Michigan Medicaid expenditures per patient with duodenal ulcer.

Further examples came from America. For instance, a classic case of medicines paying for themselves is shown in Figure 7.2. This shows that for medical expenditures in Michigan, a controlled study indicated that the use of cimetidine reduced overall treatment costs from 721 dollars per patient to 221 dollars.[4] All of these examples illustrate how modern medicines can reduce overall health service costs.

The next two examples illustrate a different point. This is the fact that a more expensive medicine may turn out to be the most cost-effective overall. Table 7.3 gives an example, again from America. This shows that using the more expensive third generation cephalosporin as a surgical prophylaxis to prevent postoperative infection would not only be more economical than using no antibiotic, but would also be cheaper overall than using a first generation cephalosporin. This is so even although the more recent antibiotic was more than twice as expensive as the older one.[5]

Turning to cancer chemotherapy, Table 7.4 shows that even although carboplatin is more than ten times as expensive as the older cisplatin, it still turns out to be the cheaper treatment because it can be given as an outpatient therapy instead of needing a stay in hospital.[6] These two examples underline the fact that considering overall 'efficiency' in terms of the cost of a medicine in isolation can often result in a less cost-effective policy being adopted.

Of course some medicines will inevitably add to total costs: they do not always result in savings. However, when the benefits are set against these additional costs the medicines may still appear to give good value for money. One example is the use of medicines to reduce cholesterol in high risk groups of individuals. The Standing Medical Advisory Committee has estimated that in the United Kingdom the extra costs of screening and medication for those

TABLE 7.3:   Savings from antibiotic prophylaxis in surgery per 100 patients

	Extra hospital cost	Cost of antibiotic	Net extra cost
No antibiotic	$707,600	—	$707,600
1st generation cephalosporin	$246,100	$5,000	$251,100
3rd generation cephalosporin	—	$11,800	$11,800

TABLE 7.4:   Comparative costs (£) for carboplatin and cisplatin

Item	Carboplatin	Cisplatin
Carboplatin 450 mg or cisplatin 100 mg	205.71	17.90
Dexamethasone iv mg + 2 mg tablets × 4 for 4 days	2.34	
Metoclopramide 150 mg iv		3.30
Domperidone tablets 20 mg × 4 for 4 days	3.47	
0.9% iv saline	0.55	3.60
Hospital bed	8.00	324.00
Registrar's time (1 hr)	8.70	
Total	228.77	347.90

recognised as being at high risk would amount to about £1,300 for each year of life through consequent reduced mortality.[7] Few people would question the fact that their next year of life was indeed worth substantially more than £1,300 to them and to their family. The *extra* health care costs from new treatments can often be justified by this sort of 'cost-utility' analysis.

Number of practices

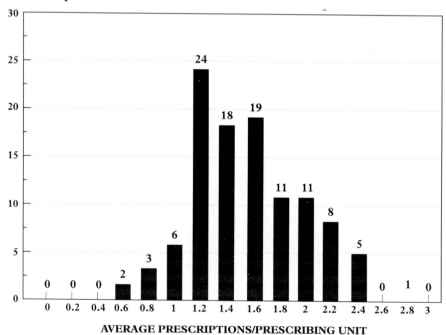

AVERAGE PRESCRIPTIONS/PRESCRIBING UNIT

Figure 7.3:   Average number of prescriptions per prescribing unit

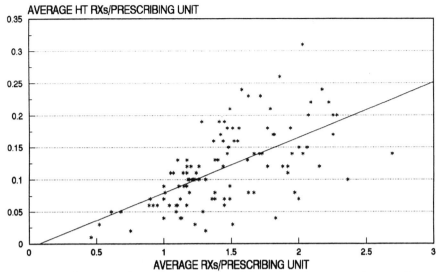

Figure 7.4: Average total prescriptions per prescribing unit against average hypertensive prescriptions per prescribing unit.

Against this background, it is relevant to examine the actual patterns of prescribing under the National Health Service. It is possible to do this using computerised data from general practices collected by the market research organisation, VAMP. The following analysis based on data from over 100 practices covers prescribing for hypertension and diabetes, for each of which diseases the actual prevalence is well established.

Figure 7.3 shows the distribution of overall numbers of prescriptions written per prescribing unit over a three-month period. Patients over 65, who are larger consumers of medicines, are scored as two 'prescribing units'. The current convention is to give these patients a score of three rather than two, but this will not significantly affect the results.

There is a cluster around 1.6 scrips per quarter – just over six per year, which accords well with data from other sources. However, the outlying extremes show a wide variation. Variation in rates of prescribing may be affected by the amounts on the prescriptions written. 'Low' prescribers may be writing scrips with larger amounts than 'high' prescribers, who may prescribe on average for very short periods.

Turning now to prescriptions written for hypertension (and specifically recorded as such in the VAMP data), Figure 7.4 shows a scatter diagram for average anti-hypertensive scrips against the average total scrips. There is a substantial spread, but a clear overall correlation ($r = 0.61$) between high total prescribing and high prescribing for hypertension, shown by the regression line on the diagram. 'High' prescribers appear to treat a larger proportion of patients for hypertension.

Figure 7.5 shows the distribution of average numbers of anti-hypertensive scrips per patient per quarter for 108 practices. Here the range between 'outlyers' is sixteen-fold – about three times as great as the range for overall prescribing. Excluding 'outlyers' the range is six-fold with an average of about 0.5 scrips per prescribing unit per year.

Number of practices

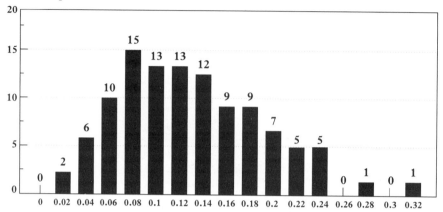

AVERAGE ANTIHYPERTENSIVE RXs/PRESCRIBING UNIT

Figure 7.5:   Average number of anti hypertensive prescriptions per prescribing unit.

On the admittedly cavalier assumption that the average prescription was for one month's treatment, this would mean that about 4% of patients were being treated for hypertension. This corresponds well with the estimate from the Royal College of General Practitioners Research Unit, which gave an estimate of 3.7% of patients treated in 1981/82.[8] It is generally estimated that the true prevalence of moderate to severe hypertension (diastolic pressure > 110 mmHg) is nearer 5%. The prevalence of hypertension above 95 mm of Hg, which the WHO recommends should be treated, is about 15%.

The estimates for numbers treated at the extremes may be significantly affected by the average size of prescriptions written, but, if the prescriptions of the lowest prescribers were for a month's treatment, it would mean that over 30% of practices are treating fewer than 3% of their patients, with the lowest prescribers treating fewer than 1% of their patients. At the other extreme, on the same assumption high prescibers may be treating most of their patients with mild to moderate hypertension (diastolic pressure > 95 mmHg).

The degree of 'underprescribing' which appears to occur among the lower prescribers is very significant in view of the increased risk of stroke among patients with untreated hypertension.[9] However, it needs to be emphasised that these data for hypertension relate to the number of prescriptions written rather than the number of patients treated.

Under-prescribing can also be demonstrated in diabetes. Figure 7.6 shows the scatter diagram relating scrips for diabetes to total scrips for the different practices. Again there is a positive correlation ($r = 0.46$) between high overall prescribing and high prescribing for diabetes. 'High' prescribers appear to be treating a larger proportion of patients for diabetes.

However, the really fascinating data come in Figure 7.7. This uses the division of prescribers into quartiles, according to their levels of overall prescribing. For insulin, there is no difference in the rates of prescribing between those who are high and those who are low overall prescribers. Both high prescribers and low prescribers write the same proportion of scrips per prescribing unit for

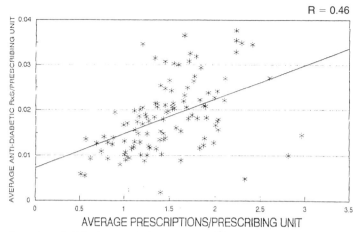

Figure 7.6: Average anti-diabetic prescriptions per prescribing unit against average prescriptions per prescribing unit.

insulin. The conclusion must be that both high and low prescribers are seeing and treating the same proportion of insulin-dependent diabetes in their practices. Early-onset insulin-dependent diabetes is, after all, a disease which is dramatic in its onset, and impossible to ignore. Its prevalence appears to be uniform between the practices.

By contrast, late-onset non-insulin-dependent diabetes is more difficult to recognise. Though many doctors screen for diabetes, there is anecdotal evidence that it is sometimes first diagnosed by an optician noting retinal damage or even by a chiropodist noting signs of peripheral vascular disease in the feet and toes. The VAMP data appear to indicate that low overall prescribers are significantly less likely to treat non-insulin-dependent diabetes than high overall prescribers. The 'intermediate-high' quartile of doctors – those with

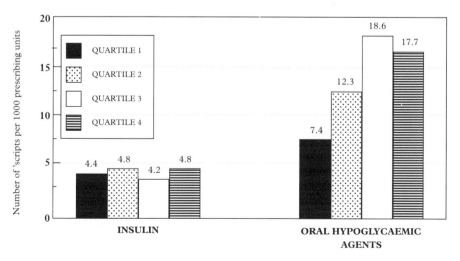

Figure 7.7: Average number of anti-diabetic scripts per prescribing unit.

TABLE 7.5:   Number of diabetic patients and prevalence per 1000 prescribing unit (PU)

	Quartile 1	Quartile 2	Quartile 3	Quartile 4
Patients treated with insulin	435	352	291	243
(Prevalence per 1000 PU)	(2.2)	(2.4)	(2.2)	(2.2)
Patients treated with oral hypoglycaemic agent	648	690	765	631
(Prevalence per 1000 PU)	(3.3)	(4.8)	(5.8)	(5.7)
Patients treated with diet alone	829	637	545	495
(Prevalence per 1000 PU)	(4.2)	(4.4)	(4.1)	(4.4)
Total prescribing unit	196,764	144,069	132,131	111,359
(Total prevalence per 1000 PU)	9.7	11.7	12.1	12.3

high, but not the highest, overall prescribing – prescribe oral antidiabetic drugs almost three times as often as the lowest quartile of prescribers.

Unlike the data on hypertension, further analysis of the diabetic data has eliminated the effects of variations in prescription size, and the results are shown in Table 7.5. This table confirms that the rate of patients treated with insulin is consistent between high and low overall prescribers. Interestingly, it also shows that the number of diabetics per thousand treated by diet alone is more or less constant between low and high prescribers.

The only variation occurs in the number of patients per thousand treated with oral antidiabetic agents. The gradient between high and low rates of treatment is less dramatic than in numbers of prescriptions, but practices in the third quartile still treat 75% more patients with oral antidiabetics than practices in the lowest quartile.

Overall, the total number of patients treated for diabetes (which is slightly higher than the number of 'prescribing units' treated) is about 13 per thousand. It has been estimated that the true prevalence of diabetes in Britain is nearer 20 per thousand[10] though not all require drug treatment. Nevertheless even the higher rates of prescribing appear to represent 'undertreatment' in relation to the probable total population of diabetic patients.

Thus not only is there evidence that prescribing is usually cost-effective, there is also evidence that at least for hypertension and non-insulin dependent diabetes some cases of the disease are not currently being treated. This not only has serious clinical consequences for the patients, but also has economic consequences for the National Health Service. It must be concluded that good prescribing is not necessarily cheap prescribing, and just as much attention should be paid to low prescribers as to high prescribers, if a truly cost-effective prescribing policy is to be implemented. Above all, in the context of NHS general practitioner prescribing, indicative prescribing amounts must be based on objectives for outcomes of medical care, and must not be based on cost considerations alone.

References

1. Teeling-Smith, G. and Wells, N. E. J. (1985). The economic contribution of the industry in England and Wales. *Pharmaceutical Journal* **235**, 178–179.

2. Griffin, J. R. (1990). *Osteoporosis and the Risk of Hip Fracture*. London, Office of Health Economics.
3. Teeling-Smith, G. (1988). *Economics of Cardiovascular Disease*. In: Postgraduate Cardiovascular Seminars. I. Ed. Sleight, London, P. Mediq Ltd.
4. Gwebe, J. and Weisbrod, B. A. (1982). *Assessing Technological Change: The Case of a New Drug*. Madison, University of Wisconsin.
5. Mandell-Brown, M., Johnson, J. T. and Wagner, R. L. (1984). Cost effectiveness of prophylactic antibiotics and head and neck surgery. *Otolaryngology Head and Neck Surgery* **91**, 520–523.
6. Tighe, M. and Goodman, S. (1988). Carboplatin versus cisplatin. *Lancet ii*, 1371–1372.
7. O'Brien, B. J. (1991). *Cholesterol and coronary heart disease*. London, Office of Health Economics.
8. Morbidity statistics from general practice. Third National Study 1981–82. (1986). Series MB5 No. 1 London, HMSO.
9. Dale, S. (1989). *Stroke*. Office of Health Economics.
10. Laing, W. A. and Williams, R. (1989). *Diabetes*. London, Office of Health Economics.

Generic Equivalence is Not a New Problem; An Example with Chloroform Dated 1849!

Dear Sir,

In answer to your request allow me to state that I have tried different varieties of chloroform made by different manufacturers; but I have always preferred yours because I have always found it the best. – I have now used several thousand ounces of the article manufactured by you; I never saw in any single case any bad effect that I could attribute to its employment. Perhaps I may add that I have seen specimens of chloroform so bad that I would be terrified to exhibit them to any patient; some of these specimens was from a large & influential London House, & of their own manufacture.

Yours very truly

A. J. Simpson

To Dr Duncan

Edinburgh 22 Oct - 1849

8   Generic Medicines: A Question of Quality

Alexander Florence

Introduction

It has sometimes proved difficult for the question of generic equivalence and inequivalence to be viewed scientifically and objectively, because of the political, professional and economic attitudes towards the increasing use of generic medicines. It is striking that many commentators view the problem as clear-cut: either generic drugs are 'inferior' and 'dangerous' or they should always be prescribed and dispensed. There is no logical way in which either stance can be defended. Some generic medicines are equivalent to the brand leader, some are not. For a given drug, several generic versions may be equivalent to a brand leader, but not all. The question, given the obvious possibility of differences in formulation and in dosage form influencing the behaviour of a medicine in the patient, is whether differences in pharmacokinetics are important enough to be of clinical concern.

Prescribers must expect that the medicines provided for patients meet the highest standards of safety, quality and efficacy. It is around the issue of quality, but sometimes also the question of safety and efficacy, that the debate on generic medicines revolves. In this chapter the term 'generic' medicine is used in the sense of a formulation of a drug, patent protection for which has expired. Generic medicines are not necessarily unbranded, many now bearing brand names, but they are to a greater or lesser extent, 'copies' of the originator's branded product. Most generic medicines are manufactured and licensed with the intention that they can be prescribed and dispensed in place of the originator's product. All generic medicines in the U.K. hold full Product Licences. Data on the drug substance, the formulation and now, almost invariably, on their bioavailability have been scrutinised by the Medicines Control Agency. Not infrequently clinical data are now furnished by manufacturers of generic medicines in support of their product licence applications. Generic medicines have at the time of licensing been considered to be equivalent both pharmaceutically and clinically and therefore to be therapeutic equivalents. This chapter will examine this claim as a general hypothesis, and will argue that identicality of product and performance can be achieved but may not always be achieved. It will not examine the many economic and other aspects of the promotion and use of generic medicines[1] some of which are laid out in Table 8.1.

Generic medicines have been around for some time and are here to stay. When patent protection on a drug substance expires, generic versions of once new chemical entities may be manufactured and sold under approved names or as branded drugs. The debate in the form 'generic' versus 'branded' medicines was never valid, because it should always have been about the clinical equivalence of products containing the same drug, whatever their source,

TABLE 8.1:   Issues surrounding generic medicines

Scientific issues

The probability of equivalence;
The probability of inequivalence;
The evidence of equivalence and inequivalence.

Medical issues

Therapeutic consequences;
Influences on patient compliance;
Substitution;
Medico-legal problems.

Political issues

Appropriate rewards for the research-based industry;
Means of controlling the drug bill;
Competition;
Effects on research investment in the UK.

Economic issues

Can economies be achieved?
At what expense?
Can we judge a product by its price?

and whether branded or unbranded. This chapter surveys the position of generic drugs in the United Kingdom, drawing on experience in other parts of the world. Since the present author attempted a review of the literature on the subject in 1972,[2] many of the new chemical entities that were marketed for the first time then, and many that had not yet seen the light of day, such as cimetidine, propranolol, ibuprofen and indomethacin, are now available as generic drugs. So there is no question, as perhaps was once the case, that the generic medicines issue relates to minor products used for relatively trivial indications. It is timely to summarise the subject, because, if anything, the situation has become more complex. Not only are the drugs that appear in generic medicines often highly potent and valuable therapeutic agents, but there is an increasing proliferation of modified release delivery systems and special formulations (such as transdermal patches), where the determination of equivalence is less straightforward.

Ensuring bioequivalence

On the one hand it could be argued that the problem of ensuring bioequivalence lies with the Medicines Control Agency (MCA), and in particular the Committee on Safety of Medicines (CSM). For this to be an effective means of guaranteeing equivalence of products in clinical use, reliance is placed on the studies presented to the CSM for licensing and on continued good manufacturing practice to ensure batch to batch reproducibility. Applications for generic products have to be scrutinised with the same rigour, often demanding those initial trials of bioavailability and experience in the clinic that are demanded from the innovator. Sometimes, licensing authorities have not considered absolute bioequivalence to be an essential requisite. In products which are variably absorbed, it is difficult to prove equivalence unless very large numbers of volunteers or patients are used in studies. The variability in the absorption characteristics of an individual drug, or the lack of correspondence between drug plasma levels and clinical effects sometimes suggests that there is little reason to insist on products producing identical plasma levels from identical doses. However, a sustainable view is that, to minimise biological variability, which might be inherent in a drug, the dosage form should be as consistent in performance as possible. The possibility of changes in clinical effect due to change of prescription from one brand to another should be minimised. It is the concern over the consistency of standards of manufacture and quality assurance and control that has to be addressed.*

There is, of course, no reason why it is not possible pharmaceutically to produce consistent generic products of conventional release tablets or capsules, or topical or parenteral formulations. For products to be essentially similar, they should contain the drug in the same amounts in the same physical and chemical form and in a similar state of purity or impurity as the brand leader, and in many cases should contain the same inactive excipients as the brand leader. It will not always be necessary for the latter to hold, if the original product is a simple formulation where the excipients are inert in both formulations. But simple formulations, such as solutions, can be deceptive, and precipitation patterns and absorption profiles of drugs administered by the intravenous route and by intramuscular or subcutaneous injection can show marked differences.

A number of medical practices have a generic prescribing policy, some without exceptions. The existence of practice formularies might overcome some problems of choice of products, and the use of patient held records, particularly those based on 'smart' cards would enable physicians and pharmacists to collect and codify data on the performance of generic products from a range of sources. The formation of the British Generic Manufacturers' Association (BGMA) seeks to counteract the effect of imported medicines and to ensure that the UK generic industry is strong.

Essential Similarity

Under European drug legislation, many generic manufacturers, in applying for product licences, claim 'essential similarity' of their product with the brand leader. The issue of 'essential similarity' of drug and product is one that was raised by the action by Smith, Kline & French over generic cimetidine,[3] although this focused on the nature of the drug substance and its impurity patterns, rather than on issues of bioavailability. Impurities can be the cause of toxic reactions,[4] as has recently been demonstrated with L-tryptophan, contaminated by an analogue during processing. While concerns have been raised in the past about poor bioavailability of generic products it is equally possible that a generic product will have a superior bioavailability to an originating brand, because of improved formulation techniques or manufacturing technology since the brand leader was marketed. This presents regulatory authorities with a dilemma and is why it is important that the formulation of new chemical entities is optimised, as today's new drugs are tomorrow's generics.

---

*These concerns are often allayed when it is clear that generic manufacturers often manufacture branded products under contract to research-based companies. Now several of the latter market their own generic products, so that concerns over provenance are unfounded.

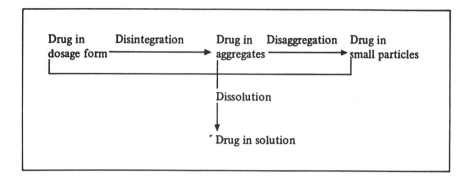

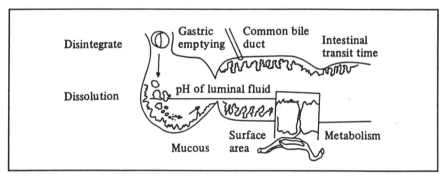

Figure 8.1: Illustrations of the processes involved in the release of a drug from an oral dosage form. In conventional tablets and capsules, disintegration into smaller aggregates precedes the solution of the drug which is then absorbed via the gastro-intestinal wall. With non-disintegrating dosage forms (such as some sustained release preparations) the process of gastric emptying may determine the absorption profile of the drug.

It is important that this whole issue is put in perspective. To that end, the potential causes of inequivalence of conventional release dosage forms, parenteral medications and specialised delivery systems will be discussed as will some of the general issues of generic substitution and inequivalence. Individual drugs will be discussed to give examples of potential problems in the clinic, and some proposals made for the future.

Equivalence of Pharmaceutical Products

The subject of therapeutic equivalence of products must be approached from a basic point of view. We must examine why products might behave differently in patients and if they do, whether or not it is important. A formulation comprises the drug plus pharmaceutical adjuvants which are generally inert (but not always in all patients[5]). The product (the dosage form) is the result of a manufacturing process varying from simple to complex; processing parameters (such as tablet compression force) can influence the performance of the product. Absorption from an oral solid dosage form, such as a tablet or capsule, involves (Figure 8.1) the disintegration of the dosage form, release of the drug and its absorption across biological membranes into the systemic circu-

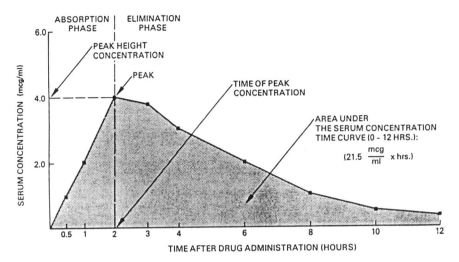

Figure 8.2: A typical serum/blood/plasma drug concentration versus time profile for a drug given orally, showing the absorption phase of the drug from the dosage form, and the elimination phase as the drug is excreted. The delivery system will affect only the absorption phase, and the resulting peak concentration (C_{max}) and the time of the peak concentration (t_{max}). The area under the curve (AUC) is frequently used as a measure of bioavailability, although it is not the sole determinant of response. C_{max}, t_{max}, and AUC must be considered together.

lation. Bioavailability is measured by determination of drug or metabolites in the blood, as the only feasible measure of availability, even though the site of action is often extravascular. There are frequently good correlations between blood/plasma levels and therapeutic effects but this is not always evident, frequently because of the complex pharmacological, metabolic and pharmacodynamic cascades that precede action.

Absorption leads to the typical blood (serum/plasma) concentration versus time profile obtained after oral, rectal, intramuscular or subcutaneous administration of a drug (Figure 8.2) from which several important features can be discerned, the peak height concentration (C_{max}) and the time of the peak concentration (t_{max}), as well as the area under the curve (AUC) as a measure of the total amount of drug which enters the systemic circulation over a given period. Often a lower threshold concentration is defined, below which clinical activity is minimal and an upper concentration above which the incidence of toxicity increases. This leads to the definition of therapeutic or optimum ranges, but these naturally vary from patient to patient, and are statistical concepts. Different products might have identical AUCs but have sufficiently different C_{max} and t_{max} values to produce different clinical effects, particularly if C_{max} (Figure 8.2) is related to side effects or t_{max} is unusually delayed so that the onset of activity is prolonged. Rates of drug release are controlled by the nature of the formulation and can often be correlated with absorption where absorption is intrinsically rapid. In other words the formulator can control release and absorption, which is the basis of controlled and sustained release products, discussed below. Different salts of a drug, even, because of different solubilities and physical properties, can influence absorption, even from liquid

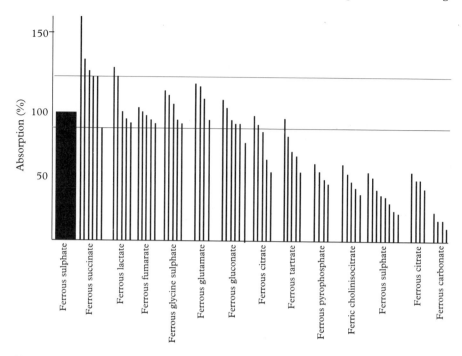

Figure 8.3:   Absorption of iron from liquid preparations, from Brise and Hallberg.[6]

preparations as the data[6] on iron salts, now nearly 30 years old, in Figure 8.3 show. Changing the tablet formulation can also alter serum drug levels, as in the (now almost classical) example of phenytoin[7] (Figure 8.4), an effect brought about by changing the effective solubility and release rate of the drug.

Patient Variability

The argument may be put forward that small differences in bioavailability between products are of little relevance because of patient variability. It is certainly clear that a given dose of the same product in different patients can produce marked variation in bioavailability. Serum salicylate levels as a marker (Figure 8.5) 3 hours after the administration of oral sodium salicylate at a dose of 35 mg/kg produces in 100 patients', serum salicylate levels ranging from about 15 μg/mL to 80 μg/mL.

Correlations between dosage and valproate serum levels[8] show a less than clear relationship, because of patient variability, although overall trends are clear (Figure 8.6). Chadwick[8] comments thus on this question: 'even in the case of long-established drugs there appears to be an over emphasis and over-reliance on so-called "therapeutic" or "optimum" ranges. There may be justification for use of such ranges when applied to a drug such as phenytoin, which possesses unusual pharmacokinetic properties and has a clearly defined toxicity syndrome. Even with such drugs, it must be realised that many patients with mild epilepsy will be controlled with serum concentrations below the accepted "therapeutic" range, and that some patients may tolerate and,

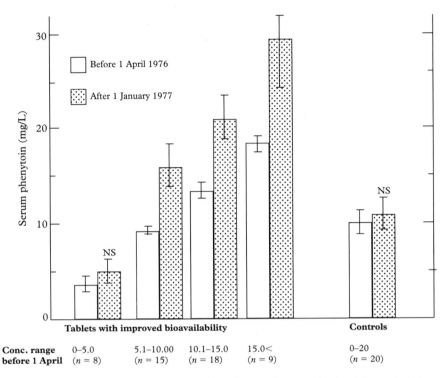

| Conc. range before 1 April | 0–5.0 (n = 8) | 5.1–10.00 (n = 15) | 10.1–15.0 (n = 18) | 15.0< (n = 9) | 0–20 (n = 20) |

Figure 8.4: The effect of change in tablet formation on the serum levels of phenytoin before and after the alterations to the formulation in 1976/1977, from Neuvonen.[7]

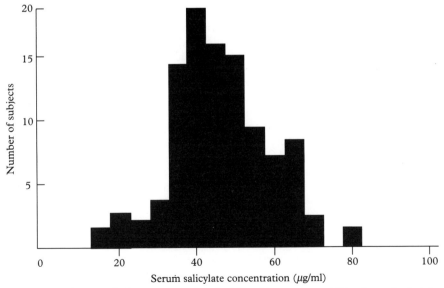

Figure 8.5: Serum salicylate concentrations in 100 subjects measured 3 h after oral administration of 35 mg/kg of sodium salicylate.

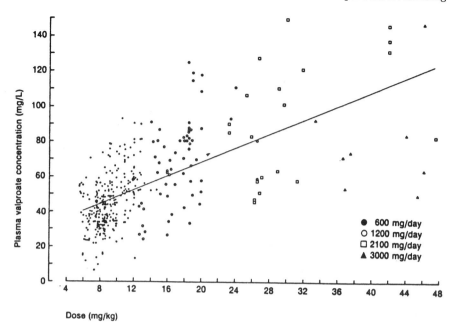

Figure 8.6: Plasma valproate concentrations (mg/L) as a function of dose (mg/kg) and dose schedule (from 600 mg/day to 3000 mg/day) showing a complex relationship, the spread of plasmal levels at each dose but the trend of increasing levels with increasing dose and daily dose, from Chadwick.[8]

indeed require serum concentrations above such ranges for adequate seizure control. The concept of "therapeutic" range becomes even more dubious when applied to a drug such as valproic acid whose plasma concentrations show considerable diurnal variation and which lacks a clearly defined syndrome of neurotoxicity. With such a drug, the most satisfactory method of monitoring its use is via its clinical effect.'

Such approaches require more extensive monitoring of patients than now occurs in general practice if we are to detect differences in products. To add to such unavoidable variability with products which are not essentially similar would appear not to be good prescribing practice.

The less variability that arises from the pharmaceutical dosage form, the less biological variability there will be. It cannot be good practice to increase variability with variable products. Obviously it is still virtually impossible to predict, in spite of the use of Bayesian pharmacokinetic evaluation of population groups, what plasma levels are going to be achieved in individuals, but a diagram such as that in Figure 8.7 can be produced to indicate the tendencies. As plasma concentrations are increased there is a therapeutic response in an increasing proportion of patients. With adverse effects which are secondary to the main pharmacological effect increasing numbers of patients will be put at risk with plasma levels increasing above the average threshold level.

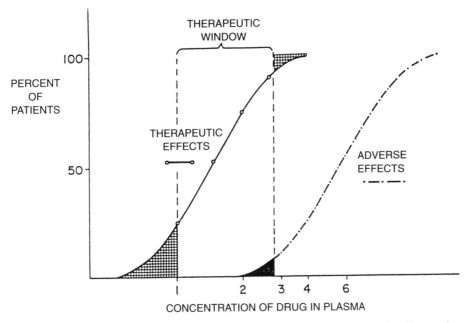

Figure 8.7: A representation of dose-response curves showing both therapeutic effects and adverse effects. The concept of the therapeutic window is partly a statistical one, as discussed in the text. In spite of variability in response to drugs, higher levels of drugs generally produce a greater likelihood of side effects, and lower levels, the opportunity for ineffective outcomes.

Generic Equivalence

Equivalence between products can be categorised at several levels: chemical equivalence, biological and clinical or therapeutic equivalence. *Chemical equivalence* is found in products containing the same amount of active ingredient in the same type of dosage form. Recent definitions of essential similarity concentrate also on the essentially similar purity of the drug substance, as well as on the release rate of the drug from the dosage form, all preludes to: *biological equivalence,* found in chemically equivalent products that produce essentially the same bioavailability, as measured by the AUC. However, the critical measure is of clinical or therapeutic equivalence of products which produce essentially the same therapeutic effects and essentially similar adverse effects. Adverse effects are, however, not always simply the result of the drug substance but will perhaps, as with the Osmosin brand of indomethacin result from a combination of drug, additive and dosage form.

Levels of inequivalence vary from clinical failure (Table 8.2) to differences in the rate of solution of the drug from the dosage form, which may or may not translate into differences in bioavailability or performance. However, differences in dissolution rate, such as those measured for varieties of carbamazepine tablets can translate into differences in peak concentration or peak time (C_{max} and t_{max}) (Figure 8.8).

TABLE 8.2:   Levels of inequivalence between medicines

Observed problem

Clinical failure;
Differences in clinical response;
Differences in side effects and toxicity;
Differences in systemic availability;
Differences in dissolution rate.
Differences in appearance.

But differences may simply be in appearance, as shown in Figure 8.9 for four brands of amitriptyline 25 mg tablets and propranolol 40 mg, that may not in any way influence performance, but may well affect those most crucial of factors – patient compliance and peace of mind. A recent report, however, describes severe urticaria in a patient given generic naproxen tablets coloured with quinoline yellow (E104) dye.[9]

Experience With Generic Medicines

A review of experience with generic products can only be derived from the literature. Reports in the medical and scientific literature are an index of the problems of generic medicines in practice, but naturally reports tend to concentrate on the incidence of generic inequivalence rather than equivalence. It is virtually impossible to provide quantitative assessments of the problems that have occurred.

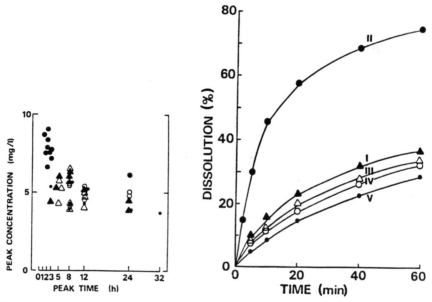

Figure 8.8:   A comparison of the peak concentrations and times to peak concentration achieved with five brands of carbamazepine. The most rapidly dissolving tablet (brand II) achieves the highest peak concentrations in the shortest times. It is this type of correlation that lends utility to *in vitro* dissolution controls (Neuvonen[11]).

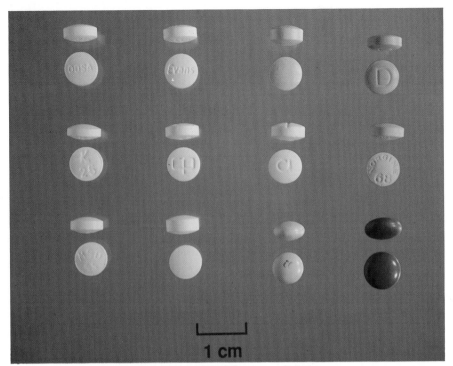

Amitriptyline   25mg

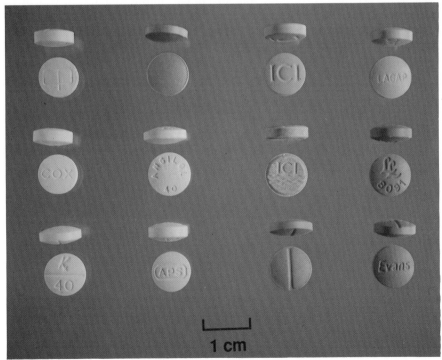

Propranolol   40mg

Figure 8.9: Photographs of different brands of amitriptyline 25 mg tablets and propranolol 40 mg tablets.

TABLE 8.3: Drugs which have been subject to bioavailability problems – The 1972 List

Acetohexamide	Oxytetracycline
Acetylsalicylic acid	Pentaerythritol tetranitrate
Aminophylline	Penicillin G
Bishydroxycoumarin	Penicillin V
Chloramphenicol	Phenylbutazone
Chlortetracycline	Phenytoin
Digoxin	Prednisolone
Erythromycin	Prednisone
Ferrous sulphate	Quinidine sulphate
Griseofulvin	Reserpine
Hydrochlorothiazide	Secobarbitone sodium
Hydrocortisone	Stilboestrol
Indomethacin	Sulphisoxazole
Isoniazid	Tetracycline
Meprobamate	Theophylline
Methandrostenalone	Thyroid
Methylprednisolone	Tolbutamide
Nitrofurantoin	Warfarin sodium

From Florence.[2]

A literature review[2] in 1972 indicated that a number of drugs had been the subject of reports of suspected and proven inequivalence (Table 8.3). Since 1972 a further list of reports can be assembled (Table 8.4). The appearance of a drug on these lists does not, of course, imply that products will be bioinequivalent, but only that there have been demonstrated the possibility of inequivalence. These are generally drugs for oral use which have a low solubility in the stomach, or whose absorption characteristics are determined by rate of release from the formulation. It is perfectly feasible to formulate and to produce consistently equivalent products of each of these substances. The

TABLE 8.4: Some instances of reported inequivalence between marketed products, post 1972

Drug	Year of reports
Aspirin	1976, 1980
Amitriptyline	1978
Carbamazepine	1985, 1987
Digoxin	1972, 1977
Frusemide	1979, 1981, 1985, 1987
Glibenclamide	1972, 1986
Glyceryltrinitrate (Tabs)	1977
(Patches)	1986, 1988
Imipramine	1979
Lithium	1974
Medroxyprogesterone acetate	1978, 1988
8-Methoxypsoralen	1977, 1980
Prednisolone	1979
Phenytoin	1974, 1975
Phenobarbitone	1982
Primidone	1987
Propranolol	1986
Tolbutamide	1975, 1985

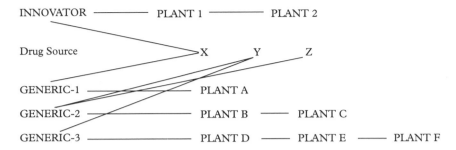

Figure 8.10: A representation of the degrees of complexity in producing reproducible drug

problem arises when individual batches from individual manufacturers some-how deviate from the specifications that have been approved in the Product Licence, set specifically to ensure equivalence and reproducibility. Each man-ufacturer has such in-house specifications for each product to ensure batch to batch reproducibility. Generic medicines are, in a way, only an extension of the batch concept to a different manufacturer. Problems are most likely to arise when the formulation of a product is critical to its performance, and where the therapeutic ratio of the drug is narrow.

Oral dosage forms have different potential for bioavailability problems as outlined in Table 8.5, solutions having the lowest potential, while complex formulations have a high potential for displaying problems. The more manu-facturers or sites that are involved in production of a medicinal product sold under a given brand name or as a generic, the greater the statistical opportu-nity for differences to occur, although, as the scheme in Figure 8.10 suggests, the finished product specification should minimise the impact of this problem. An examination, by Nightingale and Morrison[10] of 224 bioequivalence

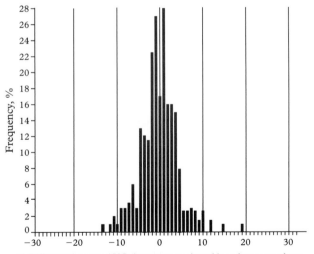

Figure 8.11: Observed differences in mean AUC's between generic and brand name products in 224 bioequivalence studies analyzed by Nightingale and Morrison.[10]

TABLE 8.5: **Relative potential of oral dosage forms to have bioavailability problems**

High	Intermediate	Low
Enteric coated tablets	Suspensions	Solutions
Sustained release	Chewable tablets	
Complex formulations	Capsules	
Slowly disintegrating tablets		

studies recorded the observed differences in mean AUCs between branded and generic products. (Figure 8.11). Very rarely did generic products deviate by more than ±10%. Various regulatory authorities will consider compliance to within ±20% to be evidence of equivalence. The AUC is, however, not the sole indicator of equivalence.

There is a dearth of literature on comparisons of UK products. Many of the examples of inequivalence used in this chapter come from the international literature and cannot necessarily be applied to the UK. But they are illustrative of the nature of the effects that are observed from time to time.

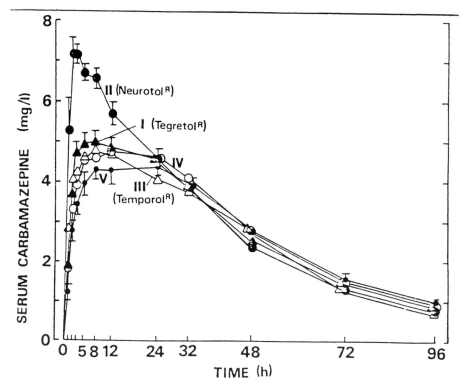

Figure 8.12: Differences in serum concentration determined after administration of five different preparations of carbamazepine, from Neuvonen.[11]

Figure 8.12 shows marked differences in peak serum levels for several Scandinavian carbamazepine products.[11] A report from the USA[12] describes breakthrough seizures in patients well controlled on Tegretol when switched to a generic carbamazepine. Differences in the rates of absorption of tolbutamide from various products has been reported.[13,14] Glibenclamide formulations have also been found in one study to display differences.[15] A correlation between diabetes control and plasma levels of sulphonylureas and biguanides has not generally been found at steady-state, and a relationship between toxic effects and drug plasma levels has only been reported for biguanides (buformin, metformin and phenformin).[16] Data on South African frusemide[17] showed differences in bioavailability and urinary output. Increased seizure frequency with generic primidone was reported in 1987 in the USA.[18]

Sometimes reports are brief and suggestive rather than conclusive, such as the report on differences in side effect incidence in patients on proprietary and generic propranolol in the UK.[19] Some are more substantial accounts. An *in vivo* study of levothyroxine brands in the US found evidence of inequivalence (between Synthroid and Levothroid)[20] leading to changes in thyroid function and clinical manifestations when patients were switched from one brand to the other. There are many reports, mainly from the USA, of inequivalence of levothyroxine tablets, some referring to differences in bioavailability and others to subpotency. In another study Synthroid tablets were compared with Levoxine brand tablets and found to be equivalent.[21] Such studies indicate the need to consider each case on its merits. It is not possible to generalise.

Differences in the efficiency of two dosage forms of 8-methoxypsoralen, (8-MOP) the photosensitizer used in PUVA treatment[22] resulted from differences in the bioavailability of the drug in the skin. One study[23] showed that the maximum plasma level achieved by one brand of 8-MOP was 5.8 times that of another (in this case an Austrian versus a Dutch product). Such differences undoubtedly affect the success of therapy, and variability in products increases the uncertainty of treatment. Marked differences in the *in vitro* release rates of the anthelmintic praziquantel from six brands of tablets were reflected, in the worst case, of the bioavailability of one generic being 70% of the brand leader[24] (study conducted in Thailand.)

Equivalence of Products for Topical and Parenteral Use

The bioavailability of many topical drugs is dictated by the formulation of the ointment, cream or gel in which it is applied. Studies by Stoughton[25] have compared triamcinolone acetonide creams and ointments using a vasoconstrictor score as a measure of bioavailability. Data shown in Table 8.6 display, particularly for the ointments, a significant difference in availability; two generic betamethasone valerate ointments were found to be equivalent to the brand leader in the same study.

Transdermal patches are sometimes promoted as if they produced a consistency of effect patient to patient. As the design and construction and indeed mechanism of release of drugs such as glyceryl trinitrate from various topical patches varies from brand to brand, so too does the release rate. AUCs for patches and ointments of nitroglycerin are given in Table 8.7, from McAllister *et al.*[26] Transiderm Nitro, Nitrodisc and Nitro-dur have been compared by

TABLE 8.6a: Triamcinolone acetonide ointments: Distribution of vasocon-striction scores by drug ($n = 30$)

Drug	Score				
	0	1	2	3	Total+
Aristocort A 0.1%	2	0	10	18	74
Goldline 0.1%*	17	12	1	0	19
Rugby 0.1%*	8	11	9	2	35

* Generic.
+ Statistical comparisons are as follows: Aristocort A is greater than Rugby ($P < .001$), is greater than Goldline ($P < .05$).

TABLE 8.6b: Triamcinolone acetonide creams: Distribution of vasoconstriction scores by drug ($n = 30$)

Drug	Score				
	0	1	2	3	Total+
Kenalog 0.1%	2	8	12	8	56
Fougera 0.1%*	8	5	15	2	41
Geneva 0.1%*	12	15	3	0	21
Goldline 0.1%*	6	13	9	2	37
Rugby 0.1%*	7	14	9	0	32
URL 0.1%*	4	16	8	2	38

* Generic.
+ Statistical evaluation of the comparisons is as follows: Kenalog is greater than Fougera ($P < .05$).
From Stoughton.[25]

Shaw.[27] At 12 h, after administration of 10 mg/24 h units, mean plasma levels ranged from 74 ng/L to 125 ng/L, the range over the period 4–24 h being circa 40 ng/L to >60 ng/L.

Injections

Formulation ingredients in intravenous, intramuscular and subcutaneous injections can affect both bioavailability and adverse reactions to the injection. Local reactions to three different formulations of diazepam when administered intravenously (a formulation in propylene glycol; a formulation containing Cremophor EL, a solubilizer; and an emulsion formulation of the drug) were dependent on formulation. Pain on injection, while not a bioavailability issue, is important for patients, and was found to be minimal with an emulsion formulation (Diazemuls).[28] In reporting an adverse reaction to etoposide (Vepesid) injection in which the patient suffered transient loss of consciousness, Donegan[29] suggests that one of the solvents, polysorbate 80, was the cause, as hypersensitivity to this agent has previously been reported. Wolff *et al.*[30] suggest that the etoposide vehicle comprising polyethylene glycol, polysorbate 80, benzyl alcohol, citric acid and ethanol, contributes to the mild disorientation observed on injection. Thus it is clear that even solutions are not necessarily simple. It is unlikely that bioavailability will be significantly different, but patient responses might well be. Essential similarity of formulations

TABLE 8.7: AUCs for patches and ointment of nitroglycerin

	Transiderm nitro	Nitro-dur	Nitrobid
Nitradisc	82.2 (64.9–104.2) NS	110.1 (86.9–138.5) NS	60.7 (47.9–76.9) $P < 0.001$
Transiderm nitro	—	133.9 (105.6–168.7) $P = 0.017$	73.8 (58.2–93.5) $P = 0.013$
Nitro-dur	74.7 (58.9–94.7) $P = 0.017$	—	55.1 (43.5–69.9) $P < 0.001$

Pairwise AUC_{0-24} ratios (%) for four nitroglycerin preparations-best estimate, 95% confidence intervals and P values.
From McAllister.[26]

for injection would avoid this problem, and declaration of ingredients on labels would assist in the identification of potential adverse reactions.

Sustained Release Formulations

Sustained or controlled release products have been designed to alter the release rate of the drug, either to reduce local and systemic toxicity (as in the case of nitrofurantoin and theophylline) or to prolong the duration of activity (theophylline). By definition sustained release (SR) products cannot be claimed to be equivalent, although some generic sustained release products might be designed to be equivalent to the brand leader and may actually be so. The UK CSM has insisted that where comparative bioavailability has not been demonstrated, generic SR products should bear a brand name to discourage substitution of one brand for another. In the case of theophylline, interchangeability between brands is restricted and patients should be retitrated when prescribed a new brand.

Pitfalls in the generic prescribing of theophylline products have been discussed in detail elsewhere.[31] Even if the therapeutic effects are similar following administration of SR products of different design, the incidence of side effects cannot be considered to be always the same. This has been shown with SR potassium chloride, lithium and theophylline. There has been a debate about the relative merits of multiple unit pelletised preparations and insoluble matrix type formulations; the latter have been associated with adverse reactions caused by their accumulation in the folds of the intestine and release of irritant molecules such as the non-steroidal anti-inflammatory drugs and iron salts over a small area of mucosa. Patients with intestinal obstructions present a special problem, and it is in such groups of patients that prescribers and pharmacists should ensure that there are no unnecessary changes in formulations dispensed.

One aspect of non-disintegrating dosage forms, as pointed out, is that their physical characteristics determine their GI transit time and their mode of interaction with food. Table 8.8 summarises the effects of food on various theophylline formulations to illustrate the formulation-dependent effects.[32]

TABLE 8.8: Summary of the effects of food on various theophylline formulations

Product	Rate of absorption	Extent of absorption
Solution	–	–
12 h preparations		
'Sabidal'	–	0
'Slo-bid gyrocaps'	– –	0
'Somophyllin CRT'	–	0
'Theobid duracap'	0	0
'Theo-dur'	– –	0
'Theo-dur sprinkle'	– – –	– – –
'Theograd'	–	+ + +
'Theolair SR'	– – –	–
24 h preparations		
'Dilatrane AP'	–	+
'Euphylong'	–	–
'Theo-24'	+ + +	+ + +
'Uniphyl'	–	+ +

Abbreviations: 0 = no effect; −/+ = slight decrease/increase (not clinically relevant); − −/+ + = moderate decrease/increase; − − −/+ + + = significant decrease/increase (clinically relevant). From Jonkman.[32]

Knowledge of Treatment

In prescribing sustained release or modified release products by brand name the doctor and patient should be able to rely on the consistency of the product, and an individual prescriber can gain experience with that product. If prescribing is generic, unless complete medication records are kept by doctor, patient and pharmacist, there will be difficulty in identifying adverse reactions and side effects which may be formulation/brand related.

The Case for Control of Generic Medicines

Because clinical measurement of therapeutic outcome is generally less secure than analytical determination, say, of plasma levels, measured blood levels are frequently compared. It is sometimes claimed that pharmacokinetic differences are of little clinical consequence, so the relationship between plasma levels and clinical outcome with drugs must be considered. It is, however, a long extrapolation to aver that, because, simple relationships between plasma level and effect can not be found, plasma levels are of no consequence. The question reverts to that of acceptable levels of variability; with a drug which is absorbed to a variable extent, and which exerts a variable clinical effect in different individuals it would seem to make sense to ensure that the input functions are as constant as possible. That is to say, that the variability due to dosage-form factors are minimised.

As and until patient-held medication records are mandatory and all concerned have the necessary data on which to base judgements on quality and performance, generic prescribing of SR products is a doubtful practice.

The situation is not so clear cut with 'conventional' release tablets and capsules which form the majority of prescribed medicines. It might be argued that as physicians can prescribe a range of doses of a drug because a product is available in more than one strength, or can effectively choose different absorption rate profiles because the medication is available as a conventional release and a slow-release product, then there can be little harm done if there are several generic products available with different bioavailabilities and different rates of absorption. If this argument is examined, it is simply an argument for the abolition of strict quality control. Whereas good pharmaceutical practice has ensured that the purity of the drug substance and the characteristics of the dosage form and the dose contained within each dosage unit, is controlled to within narrow limits at the time of manufacture and throughout the shelf-life of the product, and that each batch is consistent, the existence of one or more products which have similar but overlapping specifications has the same result as the relaxation of the specifications and standards of the original product. So the heart of the issue may be the interchangeability of generic and branded products. If the products are truly bioequivalent there can be no argument about their interchangeability. Substitution of one for the other will have little consequence.

The problem arises when there is a blanket rule or, worse, legislation which attempts to cover all dosage forms of all types of drug substance. Much depends on the rigour not only of the licensing process but subsequent inspection of manufacturing plants to ensure that original specifications and processes which are licensed are adhered to. Griffin[33] has argued that there should be several conditions under which generic medicines should be licensed (Table 8.9). These seem to be reasonable demands. If applied rigorously, then many of the problems with generics would disappear. But recent reports that manufacturers occasionally have difficulty maintaining high quality suggest that constant vigilance is required by manufacturer, pharmacist, prescriber and patient.

In conclusion, therefore, prescribers and pharmacists should always seek assurance from manufacturers about the quality of their products, their claimed bioequivalence and the consistency batch to batch if they are concerned at all about the use of generic drugs which have a narrow therapeutic ratio.

TABLE 8.9: Conditions under which generic medicines should be licensed

(1) They should have the same declared content of active ingredient as the original product marketed under a brand name;

(2) they should have the same bioavailability as the original brand named product;

(3) they should not contain any excipients that were not included in the branded product if such excipients were likely to have allergenic or toxic potential e.g. Cremophors, tartrazine or gluten;

(4) the licensing authority should ensure that generic products imported from abroad were manufactured to the same standards of GMP as required for UK-based companies.

Meeting of Pharmaceutical Trade Marks Groups, Harrogate, 1985.
From Griffin.[33]

References

1. Lamy, P. P. (1986). Generic equivalents: issues and concerns. *Journal of Clinical Pharmacology* **26**, 309–316.
2. Florence, A. T. (1972). Generic equivalence: a look at the literature. *Pharmaceutical Journal* **208**, 456–63.
3. Evans, D. J. (1952). SKF Cimetidine case. Analytical profiles of generic cimetidine products. Asian *J. Clinical Practice* Suppl. 1, 39–43.
4. Cartwright, A. C. (1990). Toxicology of impurities in organic synthetic drugs. *International Pharmacy Journal* **4**, 146–150.
5. Florence, A. T. and Salole, E. G. (1989). Adverse Reactions to Formulations. London: Wright.
6. Brise, H. and Hallberg, L. (1962). Iron absorption studies. *Acta Medica Scandinavica*, Suppl 376, **171**, 7–73.
7. Neuvonen, P. J. (1979). Bioavailability of phenytoin. Clinical pharmacokinetics and therapeutic implications. *Clinical Pharmacokinetics* **4**, 91–103.
8. Chadwick, D. W. (1985). Concentration effect relationships of valproic acid. *Clinical Pharmacokinetics* **10**, 155–163.
9. Bell, T. (1991). Colourants and drug reactions. *Lancet* **338**, 55–56.
10. Nightingale, S. L. and Morrison, J. C. (1987). Generic drugs and the prescribing physician. *Journal of the American Medical Association* **258**, 1200–1204.
11. Neuvonen, P. J. (1985). Bioavailability and central side effects of different carbamazepine tablets. *International Journal of Clinical Pharmacology, Therapeutics and Toxicology* **23**, 226–232.
12. Sachedo, R. C. and Belendiuk, G. (1987). Generic versus branded carbamazepine. *Lancet* **i**, 1432.
13. Olson, S. C., Ayres, J. W., Antal, E. J. and Albert, K. S. (1985). Effect of food and tablet age on relative bioavailability of two tolbutamide products. *Journal of Pharmaceutical Sciences* **74**, 735–739.
14. Rupp, W., Dibbern, H. W., Hajdn, P. *et al.* (1975). Untersuchungen zur bioequivalenz von tolbutamid. *Deutsche Medizinische Wochenschrift* **100**, 690–695.
15. Chalk, J. B., Patterson, M., Smith, M. H. and Eadie, M. J. (1986). Correlation between *in vitro* dissolution *in vivo* bioavailability and hypoglycaemic effect of oral glibenclamide. *European Journal of Clinical Pharrnacology* **31**, 177–182.
16. Marchetti, P. and Navalesi, R. (1989). Pharmacokinetic-pharmacodynamic relationships of oral hypoglycaemic agents: an update. *Clinical Pharmacokinetics* **16**, 100–128.
17. Meyer, B. H., Muller, F. O., Swart, K. J., Luus, H. G. and Werkman, J. M. (1985). Comparative bioavailability of four formulations of furosemide. *South African Medical Journal* **68**, 645–647.
18. Wyllie, E., Pippinger, C. E. and Rothner, D. (1987). Increased seizure frequency with generic primidone. *Journal of the American Medical Association* **259**, 1216–1217.
19. Sanderson, J. H. and Lewis, J. A. (1986). Differences in side-effect incidence in patients on proprietary and generic propramolol. *Lancet* **i**, 967–968.
20. Ramos-Gabatin, A., Jacobson, J. M. and Young, R. L. (1982). *In vivo* comparison of levothyroxine preparations. *Journal of the American Medical Association* **247**, 203–205.
21. Curry, S. H., Gums, J. G., Williams, L. L., Curry, R. W. and Wolfson, B. B. (1988). Levothyroxine sodium tablets: chemical equivalence and bioequivalence. *Drug Intelligence and Clinical Pharmacy* **22**, 589–591.
22. Polano, M. K. and Schothorst, A. A. (1977). Differences in the efficiency of two delivery forms of 8-methoxypsoralen. *Dermatologica* **154**, 216–218.
23. Andersen, K. E., Menne, T., Gammeltoft, M., Hjorth, N., Larsen, E. and Solgaard, P. (1980). Pharmocokinetic and clinical comparison of two 8-methoxypsoralen brands. *Archives of Dermatological Research* **268**, 23–29.
24. Kaojarern, S., Nathakarnkikool, S. and Suvanakoot, U. (1989). Comparative bioavailability of prasiquantel tablets. *Drug Intelligence and Clinical Pharmacy* **23**, 29–32.
25. Stoughton, R. B. (1987). Are generic formulations equivalent to trade name topical glucocorticoids? *Archives of Dermatology* **123**, 1312–1314.
26. McAllister, A., Mosberg, H., Settlage, J. A. and Steiner, J. A. (1986). Plasma levels of nitroglycerin generated by three nitroglycerin patch preparations, Nitradisc, Transiderm-Nitro and Nitro-Dur and one ointment formulation. *British Journal of Clinical Pharmacology* **21**, 365–369.

27. Shaw, J. E. (1984). Pharmacokinetics of nitroglycerin and clonidine delivered by the transdermal route. *American Heart Journal* **108**, 217–222.
28. Olsen, A. S. and Huttel, M. S. (1980). Local reactions to i.v. diazepam in three different formulations. *British Journal of Anaesthesia* **52**, 609–611.
29. Donegan, S. (1989). An unusual reaction to etoposide. *Drug Intelligence and Clinical Pharmacy* **23**,177.
30. Wolff, S. N., Fer, M. F., McKay, C. M., Hande, K. R., Hainsworth, J. D. and Greco, F. A. (1983). High dose VP-16-213 and autologous bone marrow transplantation for refactory malignancies: Phase I study. *Journal of Clinical Oncology* **1**, 701–705.
31. Florence, A. T. (1987). Sustained-release theophylline preparations: pitfalls in generic prescribing. In: *Therapeutics in Respiratory Medicine* A. J. Fairfax (Ed)., Royal Society of Medicine Symposium Series **117**, 23–32.
32. Jonkmann, J. H. G. (1989). Food interactions with sustained release theophylline preparations. *Clinical Pharmacokinetics* **16**, 162–179.
33. Griffin, J. P. (1985). reported in *Pharmaceutical Journal* **235**, 471.

9 Giving Prescribing Advice to General Practitioners

Mahendra Mashru

The General Practitioner – patient interaction is recognised as the cardinal feature of general practice and in approximately 70% of these interactions a prescription is written. Little information exists however on the clinical decision-making method used by the GP whilst searching for, and identifying, the most appropriate method of dealing with a particular problem. It is well recognised that GPs vary markedly in their approach to prescribing to the extent that one GP within a group practice may have less than 30% of his or her consultations resulting in a prescription as compared to another partner having more than 80% of his or her consultations resulting in a prescription.

Lack of a distinctive standardised practice makes the giving of advice on prescribing very difficult. For example, as GPs are not agreed on the diagnosis or management of such simple conditions as tonsillitis, it is understandable that studies in this discipline are often at great variance and as a consequence the treatment of this condition is even more at variance.

Furthermore, in giving advice on prescribing the lack of standardisation makes the advising process particularly difficult and the whole area of prescribing could become so subjective to the extent that no advice on prescribing would be appropriate. However, this is not the case as there are areas within the field of prescribing where objectivity can be applied quite effectively.

In the rest of this chapter, therefore, I will concentrate on the areas where objective advice can be given to general practitioners.

Before turning to this I will briefly discuss the framework in which advice is given. As a Family Health Service Authority (FHSA) Medical Adviser, I strongly favour an educational rather than a disciplinary approach to giving advice.

Most general practitioners wish to know how they prescribe and are keen to discover how they can do better. This climate is especially helpful to the introduction of prescribing audit. Audit is described as a review of one's own prescribing performance in a particular area as compared to a standard set either by oneself or one designed in collaboration with the Medical Adviser. Most GPs are familiar with the notion of auditing though a lot would not consider what they are doing as auditing because it is such an integral part of their work.

In a survey conducted in our FHSA area over 90% of GPs had looked at their Level 1 PACT data. In looking at the survey more closely, it was clear that most general practitioners had done some form of personal audit, and that most had established what their performance was as compared to other practices in the FHSA and nationally. They knew their average cost per item and most knew into which therapeutic group that were diverging from other GPs. Sixty-five percent of respondents stated that as a result of the internal audit they had undergone, they had altered their prescribing. In my role as a

Medical Adviser giving advice on prescribing the first task was to convey to the general practitioner that I as an Adviser in the truest sense, am to be used as someone who can be turned to for help and advice on prescribing matters; I have very little role in disciplining GPs who over-prescribe or under-prescribe. The disciplining function is carried out by another independent body set up by the FHSA, consisting of a member of the Local Medical Committee, an independent clinical pharmacologist and a representative from the FHSA who is not the Medical Adviser. In most cases this would be the Medical member of the FHSA.

When the Indicative Prescribing Scheme was introduced this was not made absolutely clear and some GPs were understandably anxious about the disciplinary role of the Medical Adviser who some GPs feared would wield power.

I was often asked as an Adviser if I was going to use my power for them or against them. I believe advisers can only work for GPs and not against GPs. There are, however, some general practitioners who still fear Medical Advisers or some that simply do not recognise that there are Medical Advisers at the FHSA. In general, when general practitioners come to know the Advisers, most have been very keen to welcome them and to use them appropriately. The other major task I had was to discover the needs of the general practitioner to enable me to respond to their needs. The major needs that were identified are dealt with below.

Needs of the General Practitioner

Soon after starting my job as Medical Adviser, I started to do various qualitative surveys on the needs of the general practitioners and from the analysis of the transcript of this survey it was obvious that most general practitioners wanted to understand PACT better and wanted to be able to come to more rational decisions as to when and what to prescribe. The full description of what PACT contains is fully contained in the chapter on 'Understanding PACT' but the summary listed below is what I go through with all general practitioners. I explain what Level 1 PACT is. If the general practitioner sounds interested I go through the Level 2 in the briefest possible manner and with a small percentage of general practitioners I go through Level 3.

There is a summary of PACT data which is useful in advising general practitioners:

Level 1 includes:

(a) Total prescribing cost for the practice.
     Total number of items for the practice.
     Cost/item for the practice.

(b) The following data are then broken down into seven sections: the six most costly therapeutic groups (cardiovascular, gastrointestinal, respiratory, musculoskeletal and joints, CNS, infectious diseases) and the rest:

     – number of items;

     – total cost;

     – average cost per item.

(c) For each doctor and the whole practice:
- list size;
- number of prescribing units (PUs);
- number of items;
- total cost;
- number of items/PU;
- number of items/patients;
- % items dispensed generically.

Level 2:

This level concentrates on prescribing costs. It is automatically sent to all practices with high costs (25% above local average).

In addition to Level 1 data, it includes:

(a) Bar charts to show the distribution of practices in the FHSA area, with the practice's own position highlighted, according to the following:
- number of items/1000 PUs;
- total cost/1000 PUs;
- average cost per item.

(b) For seven groups (the six most costly groups and all others):
- number of items and cost by section of the British National Formulary (BNF);
- leading cost drugs by BNF sub-section;
- most expensive individual drugs;
- most expensive individual preparations.

Level 3:

This can be requested by a practice or by an individual doctor. In addition to the information contained in Levels 1 and 2, the following is available:

(a) Broken down by BNF chapters:
- total cost of items;
- total number of items;
- items/1000 patients;
- cost/1000 patients;
- items/1000 PUs;
- cost/1000 PUs.

(b) Broken down by BNF paragraphs::
- quantity of each drug;
- number of prescriptions of each drug;
- total cost of each drug.

When I first started advising on prescribing not many general practitioners were interested in Level 3. However, an increasing number of general practitioners have become more interested in Level 3 than in Level 1 or 2. This is very encouraging because returning to giving advice, which is objective, it is essential to use the Level 3 PACT report. I use it straightforwardly to study such matters as the range of preparations used in a particular therapeutic group, quantities of drugs used, the prescribing rates, cost rates, average cost per item and percentage of generic prescribing.

Normally as a result of my discussion with general practitioners the desired outcome is to bring about change; I therefore spend at least the first discussion with them on their decision making style. I try to ascertain as to what and why they prescribe certain drugs and why they prescribe at all.

This initial discussion is followed by a further appointment in which I identify two or three therapeutic groups per session that we would go through. Both the general practitioner and I have to do a lot of preparation prior to this meeting and in general I request the general practitioner to get at least five sets of Level 3 PACT data. To use five sets of the data overcomes the problem of seasonal variation and also allows us to note any trends in certain drugs to show whether prescribing with a particular drug is increasing or decreasing in popularity.

During all these discussions it is essential not to lose sight of the fact that the outcome that it desired is to decide whether any change in prescribing is necessary and constantly to question why I am prescribing? Why this drug? and what am I trying to achieve? Further to this, is there a drug that I can use as an alternative which may be cheaper or more efficient than the drug I am currently using? Using this kind of thinking it is possible to bring about necessary changes in prescribing with most general practitioners. However, despite how hard Medical Advisers try there are certain concerns of general practitioners that are repeated over and over again.

I will next discuss the three main concerns that most general practitioners have reported:

Shifting the Costs of Prescribing

Cost shift is a major concern of most general practitioners who are trying very hard to stay within their indicative prescribing amounts. The NHS Management Executive recognises that there are some areas where it is unclear which doctor should most appropriately have clinical responsibility. At the interface between hospital and GP prescribing allegations of cost shift sometimes mask uncertainty about where clinical responsibility should rest.

In an attempt to delineate the extent of the problem the Management Executive is commissioning a study on this problem. Whilst we are awaiting this, most Medical Advisers are having to facilitate discussion between general practitioners and hospital doctors.

Most Medical Advisers are now included in District Drug and Therapeutic Committees to develop District prescribing policy. Some Medical Advisers seem to be making progress in this area and most importantly general practitioners are turning to Medical Advisers for help and support as they do not wish to undertake the prescribing of certain drugs which they feel ill-equipped to prescribe with a limited clinical knowledge of the drug or of resources to monitor the prescribing. Until clear guidelines are available Medical Advisers can do little more than provide support and advice where appropriate.

Another major area of concern is that of 'generic prescribing'. There are many valid arguments for and against generic prescribing and these are covered comprehensively in another chapter. I only wish to point out that generic substitution is now the rule in hospitals.

The Medicines Control Agency (MCA), formerly the Medicines Division of the Department of Health, is responsible for administering and enforcing the 1968 Medicines Act and issuing product licences. The MCA oversees the manufacture, promotion and distribution of drugs. This includes the inspection of factories both in the UK and overseas and monitoring the purity of ingredients.

The Committee of Safety of Medicines (CSM) advises on the safety, efficacy and quality of new drugs.

The Committee on Review of Medicines (CRM) has over the last 15 years reviewed the many thousands of prescriptions given 'licences of right' under the 1968 Act.

Thus both new and old drugs have been scrutinised by experts. Before issuing a product licence the MCA must satisfy itself that the drug has definable and consistent chemical properties and that it is of a specific quality and composition excluding colouring and coating. A product licence is granted if the MCA considers the drug is effective and safe. The product licence specifies the name, nature, method of manufacture and quality of medicine as well as the indications and dosages that have been approved. Any drug marketed in the UK regardless of its country of manufacture must meet specific criteria of the product licence. Doctors who claim that patients have suffered ill-effects from a generic drug have a duty to report such instances to the MCA; as an Adviser I hear many general practitioners expressing their concerns about generic prescribing and when specifically asked whether such reporting had taken place not many doctors had actually done so. It seems as though many doctors use the argument of inferior quality as a reason for not prescribing generically although this argument may be ill-founded; as Medical Adviser I see my role is to put this argument in its true perspective.

The other concern about generic prescribing is the worry about colouring that some general practitioners mention in my discussions with them. A survey of community pharmacists has shown that the complaints by patients about the colour of drugs seem to have gone down dramatically since the time the limited list was introduced. In the majority of cases patients are reassured once they are told by the pharmacist that the medicine is the same as they used to have previously but that it is made by another manufacturer.

In view of this I feel as a Medical Adviser confident in advising general practitioners to shift to generic prescribing in many circumstances. Especial care must be taken, however, in patients with epilepsy, and certain other conditions. For patients on carbamazepine and phenytoin direct switch is not possible due to differences in bioavailability and due to the nature of epilepsy where small changes in drug levels can make a significant difference to the condition. This does not, however, mean that substitution can never take place with these two drugs. All it means is that the dose would have to be retritrated if a change of medication is desired. However, in the cases of almost all the other drugs a direct switch can be made without having to retritrate. Most

GPs are becoming increasingly confident about generic prescribing and this is reflected in the fact that there is a steady increase over the years in generic prescribing. Some practices have generic prescribing of over 80% and claim that none of their patients have come to any harm as a result of this. This has obviously saved a considerable amount of money which can be used more wisely for other National Health Service activities. Chapter 8 deals comprehensively with the quality of generics.

Reduced Autonomy of General Practitioners

This is my final concern. General practitioners often query: 'Am I no longer allowed to prescribe expensive medication without asking the Medical Adviser?' In my personal opinion, the indicative prescribing amount does not reduce the autonomy of doctors as the decision to prescribe still remains with the general practitioner. The autonomy of doctors was reduced when the limited list was introduced as the list specifically dictated that certain drugs could not be used. An alternative to the indicative prescribing scheme could have been extension to the limited list and this option has still been left open. If the latter option were taken then this inevitably would lead to reduced autonomy.

Personally, both as an Independent Medical Adviser and as a general practitioner, I feel that we are still free to prescribe whatever medicines our patients need. This view is shared by most general practitioners with whom I have discussed the indicative prescribing scheme. Most Medical Advisers are competent enough to understand that there will always be variations in prescribing patterns and practice levels to take account of the type of patient and the legitimate professional preference of individual doctors. PACT was developed essentially as an educational tool and may doctors have found it helpful when undertaking self-audits of their prescribing. The Medical Advisers are there to be used to allow this educational exercise to be utilised to its full potential.

In giving prescribing advice to general practitioners I work as a mentor. I see myself as a person who helps the general practitioner to make more informed choices when he prescribes. I hope I stimulate educationally the general practitioners into thinking about what and why they prescribe. The outcome I would like to see is that every time a general practitioner puts a pen to prescription pad he or she goes through a few routine questions: is prescribing the most appropriate choice of management for this patient? Is the medicine I am choosing the most appropriate one for this patient? Is there an alternative medicine which is just as effective but which would cost less? Finally, do I know all about the medicine that I need to know, and if not should I be turning to someone for advice?

10 The Role of the Regional Health Authority in Primary Care Prescribing

Alastair Hepburn

The role of the Regional Health Authority (RHA) in Primary Care Prescribing is a new one. Before assessing this role, it is helpful to look at a simple plan of the structure of the National Health Service as recently implemented in England (Figure 10.1).

For the first time, regions have direct responsibility for Family Health Service Authority (FHSA) activities and have had to adapt fairly rapidly to an unfamiliar environment. There was an inherent danger that because of the pace of the NHS reforms, over emphasis on the purchaser/provider split and contracting issues, primary care might have been rejected to the sidelines. Fortunately this has not happened for a variety of reasons:

1. Directors of Public Health are the lead players in developing health strategy and policy and are well aware of the significance of primary care in the 1990s.

2. A new breed of FHSA general manager has ensured that they are not 'short changed' and tend to keep region on its toes.

3. The NHS Management Executive (NHSME) has made it quite clear that the focus must be on primary care – documents such as *Integrating Primary and Secondary Care*,[1] *FHSAs: Todays and Tomorrows Priorities*[2] and the government consultation paper *The Health of the Nation*[3] have repeatedly emphasised that general practice is no longer the poor relation of the hospital sector.

The Operational Role of the Regional Health Authority

The Primary Care prescribing role of the RHA can be summarised as follows:

1. allocation of firm budgets to FHSAs;

2. allocation of prescribing budgets to fundholding general practitioners;

3. monitoring the indicative prescribing scheme (IPS) using expenditure statements from the Prescription Pricing Authority (PPA) for both firm budgets, indicative prescribing amounts (IPAs) and fundholding prescribing budgets;

4. communication with the Department of Health and the FHSAs within the region both on quantity and on quality of prescribing;

5. addressing the problems which arise at the primary/secondary care interface and the production of prescribing protocols to aid this process.

91

SECONDARY CARE   PRIMARY CARE

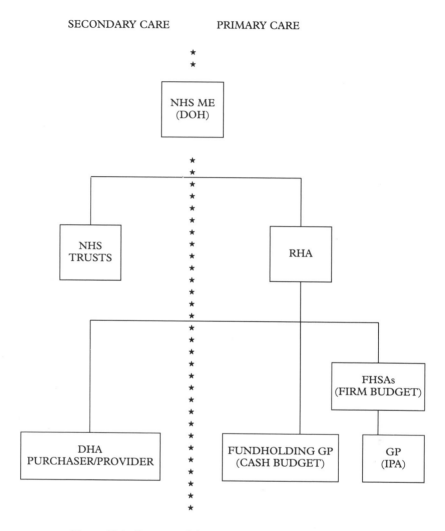

Figure 10.1: Structure of the National Health Service in England.

Firm Budgets

The firm budget is the amount required for anticipated expenditure on all pre-scriptions dispensed by community pharmacists, dispensing doctors and appliance contractors. This budget amounts, for example, to almost £290 m for 1991/92 for the two Thames regions for which I have responsibility – North West Thames and South West Thames. This figure is based on a Department of Health model which takes into account historic expenditure, demographic changes, product mix and drug inflation forecasts. The sum is *not* cash limited. There can be no virement to other areas of RHA expenditure. If the predictive power of the model proves to be inaccurate, or just cause for exceeding the firm budget can be given, reassurances have been given and continue to be given that extra funding will be made available.

At this stage, there is no evidence that any region has altered the FHSA allocation as notified by the Department of Health. Currently, there is insufficient information to do so and it will only be in future years that the accuracy of the data can be determined.

Indicative Prescribing Amounts

The key to indicative prescribing lies with the indicative prescribing amount (IPA): this is the estimated amount of annual expenditure which each general practice has allotted to it after the FHSA medical adviser has considered the various factors relevant to that practice. This is not a cash budget and there are no savings to be made or potential bankruptcies to ensue. The indicative prescribing amount is simply a benchmark against which the practice prescribing can be measured. The RHA is responsible for ensuring that these amounts have been set correctly and that the FHSA is monitoring them judiciously. The regional health authority monitors the practice aggregated FHSA indicative prescribing amounts on a month by month basis. In the unlikely event of excessive prescribing by a GP and that doctor does not respond to corrective action by the FHSA Medical Adviser, then an FHSA professional committee may find that GP in breach of his or her terms of services. The GP has the right of appeal to the regional health authority against both finding of fact and level of withholding.

RHA Strategic Role

Now that the indicative prescribing scheme is underway, regions will be increasingly involved in prescribing strategies. The most important work will include linkage of prescribing patterns with demographic and morbidity data as measurements of health status and health needs become apparent. The question that will be increasingly raised is 'does prescribing match the needs of the community?'

Inter-FHSA variation in prescribing patterns and trends will also be on the agenda as well as differences in drug utilisation. The uptake of new products introduced to the market, especially if they are likely to have a major impact on budgets, will be monitored.

Cost benefit studies will undoubtedly become more sophisticated and hopefully will be subject to independent assessment. Such studies are likely to be increasingly important when regions are sending out messages to their FHSAs on quality, efficacy and cost of prescribing.

RHA Structure

All regions have set up steering groups or similar bodies to advise on the new prescribing role. These groups tend to be multi-disciplinary with variable representation from FHSA (General Manager, Medical Adviser), DHA (General Manager, District Pharmaceutical Officer), general practice and relevant regional personnel (Regional Medical Adviser, Regional Pharmaceutical Officer, Primary Care Manager). Both operational and strategic items are likely to be on the agenda.

Operationally, the lead player at region is likely to be the Regional Pharmaceutical Officer or more rarely the Primary Care Medical Adviser.

Regional Objectives

These will depend on the RHA but my personal objectives are as follows:

1. to develop RHA policy on the equitable allocation of drug budgets to FHSAs, taking account of national guidelines and local circumstances;
2. to act as a resource for FHSAs on preparation and implementation of the indicative prescribing scheme;
3. to oversee and co-ordinate the work of the medical advisers employed by FHSAs in the two Thames regions with which I am involved;
4. to establish a forum for the exchange of views and information between the FHSA medical and pharmaceutical advisers;
5. to monitor firm budgets and indicative prescribing amounts;
6. to assess additional funding requirements and present these to the Department of Health;
7. to advise and encourage FHSAs and general practitioners to adopt prescribing policies which are:
   (a) effective;
   (b) safe;
   (c) appropriate to the needs of the patients;
   (d) economic.
8. to address the current problems at the hospital/primary care interface;
9. to encourage practice prescribing formularies;
10. to analyse FHSA prescribing patterns and variations:
    (a) at macro level;
    (b) at therapeutic group/sub-group level;
    (c) at individual drug level.

The FHSA Medical Adviser

The majority of doctors employed as FHSA Medical Advisers have been recruited from General Practice and approximately 60% are working full-time. For some, this proved to be a culture shock, brought about by the transition from independent contractor status to employees of a corporate body, with direct managerial responsibility to a General Manager. Initially the Medical Advisers tended to be somewhat isolated but inevitably they are developing a less fragmented outlook as they come under the umbrella of either their national organisation (the Medical Advisory Support Centre) or as local groups are formed. From a regional point of view, it is helpful to have regular meetings of medical advisers so that local difficulties can be discussed, policies can be devised and the various messages from the centre disseminated.

Because these doctors are a valuable and expensive commodity, their remit is normally much wider than indicative prescribing issues. The FHSA needs medical input on wide ranging topics and expert advice is crucial. Occasionally, the prime reason for their appointments – the setting up and monitoring of indicative prescribing amounts – is liable to be hijacked by other 'more interesting' topics.

Many FHSAs rely on part-time advice from GPs who are still practising. Though some FHSAs have expressed a preference to have different advisers for different tasks, others have found part-time advice to be the only solution following failure to recruit full-time doctors. The reasons for such a failure were multi-factorial but included:

1. salaries which contrasted poorly with the average earnings of general practitioners;
2. lack of career structure;
3. poor publicity from medical colleagues, press and other sources; views were often expressed that medical advisers were simply FHSA policemen.

Nevertheless, despite all these negative points there are many highly qualified medical advisers in post and as their role evolves, so they will become an increasingly powerful body. It is likely that their work will focus on the quality of primary care in their patch.

Pharmaceutical Advisers

Pharmaceutical advisers tend to be more common where the FHSA has only part-time medical advice. The job description varies, but usually involves analysing and interpreting PACT data, briefing the medical adviser before practice visits and input into local prescribing bulletins. More rarely this adviser is responsible for practice visits and, over a period of time, will have targetted all the FHSA practices to discuss their own individual PACT analysis.

Pharmaceutical advisers have a valuable contribution to make and there would undoubtedly be more in place, were it not for cash constraints at FHSA level. The majority have a district pharmaceutical service background.

Fund-Holding Practices

Indicative prescribing amounts are set for fund-holding GPs by the FHSA Medical Adviser in the same way as for non fund-holders. After the amount is agreed with the practice, the indicative prescribing amount is converted to a cash sum (approximately 9% less), to take into account pharmacist discount and container costs. The cash is subtracted from the FHSA firm budget and is transferred to the practice as part of its overall budget.

The GP fund-holder can vire money from prescribing to the other two elements of his fund – for staff and hospital costs. As the practice is able to retain savings at the end of the year, there is a clear incentive to ensure that prescribing is cost effective. This does not necessarily mean cheap. The practice may generate considerably more savings by keeping a patient out of hospital than by withholding drug therapy, even though this may be expensive. A particular problem which the regional health authority may have to face with fund-holders is the fact that the prescribing element of the fund has been transferred from a non-cash limited to a cash-limited budget. Every practice is in a constant state of flux with list sizes which are subject to unpredictable change. It is therefore apparent that if a fund-holding practice has a sudden legitimate and clinically justifiable increase in costs, this will need to be met. The practice and FHSA would need to investigate all elements of the fund to look at expenditure profiles and changes. If there are no compensating factors, the RHA will need to top up the practice budget from a contingency fund. Thus there will be no disadvantage to a fund-holding general practitioner to take on their list new 'expensive' patients.

General Practitioners

The general practitioner, with the exception of fund-holders, has little direct dealing with region (other than through its professional advisory committees). Indicative prescribing matters, controlled drugs, and border line substances, all lie within the province of the FHSA. Nevertheless, regional health authorities may receive feedback that some practices are unhappy with the way their indicative prescribing amount has been negotiated and with the fact that they had not received a visit from the Medical Adviser before the indicative prescribing amount was set. The fact that many Medical Advisers were appointed too late to visit the majority of practices was the main cause, and initially effort was concentrated on practices that were outliers when compared with the FHSA average. By the end of 1991, however, the target for all FHAs should be 100% of practices visited.

Unfortunately, the indicative prescribing scheme was implemented at the end of many contractual changes and because the concept of prescribing amounts and firm budgets is not easy to grasp, a great deal of misunderstanding persisted amongst GPs about the scheme. The situation is not aided by residual resentment over what is generally regarded as an imposed contract. The clear message from the *Improving Prescribing* document published by the Department of Health[4] that patients would be able to get all the drugs that they need, including high cost medicines, has not always been appreciated. It has been overshadowed by implications of budgetary restraint.

Department of Health

A Department of Health/Regional Liaison Group has been formed with members drawn from civil servants responsible for implementing the prescribing scheme and the lead player from each region. This has been valuable in exchanging views and alerting the Department to potential pitfalls. Various amendments and operational details of the scheme have surfaced and been discussed, though it must be said that the Department is not always receptive to the views expressed.

The Prescription Pricing Authority

The operation of the indicative prescribing scheme is dependent on the quality of information from the Prescription Pricing Authority (PPA) in

Newcastle. From this source the regional health authorities receive statements on a monthly basis for the firm budget indicative prescribing amounts for fund-holding GPs, which they hold themselves. Regions also have available on request prescribing analysis and cost (PACT) reports for each FHSA for all three levels every quarter. The details of this scheme appear in Chapters 2 and 4.

The PPA deserves a great amount of credit for the way in which it has adapted to produce this wealth of data. The main drawback is that the information is paper based and must be responsible for the destruction of many forests. Ways of transmitting data electronically are the subject of a number of pilot studies and is likely that computer links will be set up between the PPA and FHSAs.

Formularies

The pharmaceutical industry not unnaturally expresses great concern about the possible growth in the use of primary care formularies. My own view is that formularies should be practice based and drawn up by the doctors themselves using a pharmacist facilitator if required. The principal reason why practice formularies have not taken off is that GPs are currently overwhelmed with other types of paperwork relating to their new contractual arrangements. Nevertheless I would expect that FHSAs would be encouraging practices to look at prescribing protocols or formularies and taking note of the local hospital formulary.

I do not feel that there is any place for a regional formulary for general practice at present.

The Primary/Secondary Care Prescribing Interface

This issue has involved a huge expenditure of time and effort.

The Department of Health guidelines which were issued in February 1987 on prescribing responsibility stated quite categorically that the duty of prescribing for a particular element of a patient's treatment rested with the doctor who at the time had clinical responsibility for that element of care.

The decision as to which doctor has clinical responsibility for any particular aspect of the patient's treatment was for the doctors themselves to decide. It became apparent that more and more hospitals with cash limited budgets saw the primary care sector as one solution to their problems. Savings could be made by reducing or even ceasing outpatient prescribing, reducing medication given to patients discharged from hospital, and requesting GPs to take on prescribing of expensive medication (with which they may be unfamiliar).

Historically, the three major items cost-wise were:

(a) growth hormone;

(b) erythropoetin;

(c) peritoneal dialysis fluid;

Not unnaturally GPs resented this situation because:

1. they saw clinical responsibility resting with the hospital consultant;

2. if they signed the prescription form they had legal liability if problems ensued with the drug;

3. there were communication difficulties with many consultants who simply did not give the GP enough information about the patient or the drug that was expected to be prescribed;

4. they expressed concern about exceeding their indicative prescribing amounts;

5. there were worries that patients were being used as pawns in a financial chess game and that they might have to forego treatment.

Some consultants were either unaware or seemingly oblivious to the fact that their GP colleagues regarded hospital shifted prescribing as a great issue. From their point of view, if their hospital imposed a veto on the prescribing of certain drugs, there was little action they could take. A prescription issued would simply not be dispensed.

The result was that many GPs complained of moral blackmail, though most of them succumbed to pressure and prescribed the drugs for their patients so that they were not deprived of necessary treatment.

The Department of Health is issuing revised guidelines to those which have now lapsed, though the basic problem may remain insoluble. When there is no virement between budgets which are essentially of different nature, there will always be a temptation to off-load prescribing onto the primary care sector. This will be overcome to a certain extent by the new contracting arrangements between purchasers and providers when a certain level of discharge prescribing should be one of the specifications. However, if there were to be any major change of central policy on this issue, there would be a clear risk of upsetting the steady state in year one of contracting, which would cause unforeseen and possibly major difficulties.

The Pharmaceutical Industry

There have been major variations in the way in which the pharmaceutical industry has reacted to the new environment. Some companies have set up large NHS liaison units whilst others are awaiting events before entering the fray. It is nevertheless apparent to even the recidivists that the regions and the FHSAs will have an increasing influence on primary care prescribing. GPs will soon have much more drug information than previously, including comparisons of their own prescribing patterns with those of colleagues and the FHSA. They are likely to be made aware of therapeutic areas where an increase in prescribing is necessary as well as areas where there is obvious waste.

GPs will increasingly have expectations that the industry representative will be better briefed before visits and may be able to target the promoted product to the true needs of the practice population. As well as details of therapeutic advances and cost benefits, a very large degree of honesty and credibility is a pre-requisite if the GP/industry representative relationship is to flourish. Pharmaceutical sponsorship – for instance, in the field of health promotion or staff training – is often greatly valued and appreciated. Doctors for their part have a role in making companies aware of their own needs, and those of their patients. Regional epidemiological data will be required to identify shortfalls in the provision of care.

At the regional level it is also mutually beneficial to establish a dialogue with the appropriate personnel from pharmaceutical companies. Regions need to be aware of products that are likely to influence or change prescribing practice. Companies require to be alerted to the not infrequent changes of prescribing policies that may reflect on their activities. The market place is a rapidly changing environment.

Conclusion

There is a risk in becoming bogged down with the intricacies of monitoring budgets and of losing sight of the ultimate objective of the new role that has been given to regions. This is to ensure that prescribing is safe, efficacious, cost-effective and matching the needs of the population. A considerable amount of effort will be needed. One major task will be to devise outcome measures which will truly evaluate the influence of medicines on the disease process. The success of this venture is unlikely without the co-operation of all the protagonists.

References

1. NHS Management Executive (1990). *Integrating Primary and Secondary Health Care*. London, HMSO.
2. Foster, A. (1991). *Today's and Tomorrow's Priorities*. London.
3. HM Government (1991). *The Health of the Nation*. London, HMSO.
4. NHS Management Executive (1991). *Improving Prescribing*. London, HMSO.

11   Information to Doctors about Medicines: Supporting the Advisers

Gordon England

Although they have received less publicity than many of the other changes presently taking place within the National Health Service, those contained in the working paper *Improving Prescribing*[1] may ultimately be seen to be of seminal importance.

It is perhaps surprising that so little emphasis has been given historically to the wider issues surrounding prescribing by general practitioners (as opposed to individual drug studies) given that almost 50% of the total expenditure in primary care goes on drugs and that a recent survey suggested that well over 60% of GP – patient encounters result in the issuing of a prescription.

Like many subjects clinical pharmacology usually achieves only a moderate time allocation in the crowded undergraduate medical curriculum so that doctors obtain much of their expertise in prescribing during their hospital, or practice training. As Nicholas Hough has described in Chapter 3 there is also a wide range of written material available and this is supported by a variety of high quality postgraduate seminars many of which are supported by the pharmaceutical industry.

The challenge presented to the general practitioner in deciding whether and what to prescribe is arguably greater than that of his hospital colleagues in that the time available for consultation and examination is shorter, diagnostic information is less readily available, and opportunities for observations of outcome, compliance, adverse reactions and so on, are highly limited. Nevertheless, it is generally accepted that overall standards are high although the title of the working paper *Improving Prescribing* clearly indicates that the Department of Health's expert advisers considered that things could be better still. The medical literature contains many references (often based on relatively small studies) which suggest that prescribing both in primary care and in hospitals can at times be described in the Department's terms as 'wasteful or inappropriate' and the substantial variability which analysis of the PACT data set has revealed, is, at prima facia level at least, greater than seems explicable on clinical grounds.

'Improvements' in prescribing or in any other sphere can only be achieved as a result of a series of linked actions which include the definition and setting of standards, an analysis of the existing situation, the identification of those areas in which improvements might be achieved, and the establishment of a system to monitor and measure outcomes. Earlier chapters have described a variety of activities which are important components of this process and in this chapter we will consider the role which the Medical Adviser may play in the completion of the chain.

It is not often that a new speciality arises within the medical profession. It is a matter of speculation whether the appointment of FHSA Medical

Advisers with a special interest in prescribing arose as a result of analysis of need, inspiration or serendipity. What is already quite clear is that the transformation of the old FPCs into FHSAs, and the introduction of the indicative prescribing scheme, would have been almost impossible without them.

The Department recognised from the outset that the magnitude of the task facing the newly appointed Medical Advisers was such that without some form of supporting organisation it was unlikely that their efforts would be effective. Funding was therefore made available to set up the National Medical Advisers Support Centre (MASC) which together with the Medicines Resource Centre (MeReC) and the Prescribing Research Unit in Leeds provides resources to assist the advisers in implementing the aims and objectives set out in *Improving Prescribing*. The centre is located in Liverpool adjacent to MeReC to ensure a close working relationship between the two units. It is staffed by three doctors whose specialist interests include clinical pharmacology and therapeutics, postgraduate education in general practice, epidemiology, research methodology, clinical teaching, computerised data analysis and expert systems. Supporting staff include a social scientist, a health economist and a medical statistician.

Links with outside bodies such as Universities, Research Foundations and Management Training Institutes are considered important and are being developed rapidly.

There are at present (November 1991) 124 FHSA Medical Advisers in post, 47 of whom hold full-time appointments. Nationally this amounts to 7.5 sessions per FHSA or some 700 working sessions per week, a number which clearly falls far short of what is required.

Most come from a background in general practice, many from positions of some prominence with a wide range of special interests such as education, medical politics, public health, GP research and audit. The age distribution is interestingly bimodal with maxima at 41–45 and 56–60 years.

Many reasons were given in answer to the question 'why have you become a Medical Advisers?' including interest in a new challenge, frustration with general practice, a desire to become involved in management, early retirement but a feeling that they still had something to contribute, and particularly, in the younger age group, an expectation that the position might be developed into a career of considerable influence and status. Most saw the advisers' role as important and recognised that their previous experience as general practitioners taken together with new skills potentially gave them the chance to change practices within the primary care sector working at 'doctor to doctor' level.

Although in *Improving Prescribing* reference was made to 'prescribing medical advisers' it has rapidly become clear that this limitation is not practicable at operational level so that to a greater or lesser extent most advisers work as generalists. Nevertheless, 65 out of 122 listed prescribing as their principal responsibility (including the majority of those holding full-time posts) and a further 22 listed 'everything' which presumably includes prescribing. Audit, Health Promotion, Health Needs Assessment, and Budget Holding were high on the list of other activities.

The immediate tasks which confronted most Medical Advisers centred around the introduction of the indicative prescribing amount scheme and highlighted the need to acquire presentational and negotiating skills, a detailed understanding of the PACT system and some knowledge of the interaction and responsibilities of District and Regional Health Authorities. Those involved with fund holding practices also needed to understand the purchaser–provider system. These requirements determined the activities of the support centre during the initial phase of its existence. It also quickly became clear that there was a need to provide a forum in which Medical Advisers could meet together in order to exchange ideas and experiences so a number of three-day national meetings have been organised in addition to the specific skills presentations which have been provided locally in several regions. Use has been made of established providers such as universities, management schools and commercial units to run those courses which it is not economical to provide in-house.

To retain credibility, those Medical Advisers with a special interest in prescribing will need to gain considerable expertise in clinical pharmacology and therapeutics. The support centre's initial programme will concentrate on topics of major clinical interest and will be spread over a period of 12–18 months. Teaching methods are largely tutorial based but also include written material, slides and at a later stage video presentations. Co-ordination with the MeReC Bulletin is important and will be achieved whenever circumstances allow. As results become available from the Prescribing Research Unit these will be incorporated into the teaching material. The ability to assess the validity and importance of published material is also vital and specific teaching modules are part of the pharmacology programme.

To avoid unrealistic intrusion into the limited time available to advisers, distance learning packages are being developed for those interested in descriptive and analytical statistics, the elements of health economics, basic information technology and computer techniques, and the role of the specialist in public health medicine. The Department of Health has also funded research into computerised analysis and presentation of PACT and other prescribing data to facilitate the task of monitoring and improving prescribing at FHSA level. David Archer is the leader in this field and we anticipate that his work will be extended to make the analysis of PACT data more directly relevant to the needs of the Medical Advisers and more user friendly.

Whilst the main objectives of the various initiatives described in this book lie mainly in the future, certain areas are already becoming prominent as likely major determinants of success or failure.

Much emphasis has been given recently to the concept of 'value for money' or health economic evaluation in relationship to improving prescribing. Although certain well known centres of excellence such as York University and the Office of Health Economics are responsible for a significant number of publications which address this topic, it is acknowledged that the subject is relatively new and is therefore evolving. The pharmaceutical industry has responded rapidly and presentations based on economic arguments are becoming more common. The evaluation of these present considerable difficulties even to those trained in health economics and the centre will be placing some emphasis on this subject during the latter part of the year.

Perhaps the greatest challenge for the future lies around the use of new powerful drugs with highly specific modes of action or the extended use of existing therapies in response to health promotion clinics or other essentially preventative strategies. The correct balance between therapeutic advantage, risk and cost may be difficult to quantify. Experience suggests that new drugs are often used to a greater extent than their licensed indications imply or that diagnostic criteria may be difficult to apply in the primary care setting. Thus whilst a cost benefit analysis of a new form of treatment may be highly positive when it is used in accordance with the appropriate protocol (and therefore constitutes improved prescribing) the overall benefit may be reduced or even become negative as a result of inappropriate use.

Recent research in America has confirmed that direct peer contact is the most effective strategy for improving prescribing standards. The Medical Adviser is potentially therefore critical in controlling and making the best use of the many advances in therapeutics which are likely to be introduced during the next decade. This is of course sensitive territory. Doctors traditionally defend their freedom to prescribe vigorously and any action which might be interpreted as an attempt to restrict this freedom even when mediated through a medical colleague is likely to be counter-productive.

A further dimension which will require exploration is the relationship between the prescriber and the pharmaceutical industry. If the initiative to improve prescribing is to succeed it is important that the NHS and industry develop a modus vivandi that is constructive rather than simply competitive. Increased expenditure on drugs in the health service depends upon clear clinical and economic evaluations; failure to achieve this may result in some future system of arbitrary restriction such as those already introduced in other countries. It seems probable that such action would benefit neither the patient nor the pharmaceutical industry. MASC believes it has a central role to play in the development of an appropriate relationship between FHSA Medical Advisers and industry. A dialogue is already developing between the centre, Medical Advisers, the ABPI and a number of major companies which has great promise.

The appointment of Professor Michael Peckham as NHS Director of Research and Development offers many exciting possibilities for research in the primary care sector. Prescribing is a field which may well be high on his agenda and the availability of medically qualified field workers in the form of FHSA Medical Advisers when linked to the output from the Prescribing Research Unit and others engaged in similar research would potentially allow rapid progress to be made.

MASC is the natural forum in which these concepts can be debated and developed and we will be able to provide training in research methodology for those advisers who become involved in local research projects.

Medical Advisers are here to stay. During the next few years their role will expand in scale and diversity in parallel with the changes in primary care which result from the recent reorganisation. Prescribing will always be high on the agenda although it seems possible that it may develop within a speciality role. It is important to remember that prescribing is not an activity which exists in isolation.

The clinical history, examination, diagnosis and assessment of the patients psyche and circumstances are all essential preliminaries before a doctor reaches the point of deciding which, if any, drug or therapy is most appropriate and cost effective.

Improved prescribing is likely to prove quite difficult to define and even more difficult to measure, but since success would provide significant benefits to our patients, it is a challenge we are happy to accept.

Reference

1. NHS Management Executive (1991). *Improving Prescribing.* London, HMSO.

12   Formularies and Their Use

Peter Lumley and Frank Wells

Introduction

The concept of a formulary to enable prescribers to know what medicines are appropriate and available is not new. Medicines have, after all, been used for centuries. Most apothecaries and hospitals had their own special remedies and recipes, derived from plant and animal extracts, which they closely guarded. Although any similarity between the recipe books was purely co-incidental, these books were classic early examples of formularies.

History of the Development of Formularies

In the United Kingdom, it was not until 1864 that any attempt at uniformity was made. Then, the General Medical Council, which had been established six years previously, was authorised to prepare the British Pharmacopoeia. This laid down legally enforceable standards for the quality of medicines. That, however, was not enough, and a demand arose from doctors and pharmacists for more information about medicines, as many of the preparations then available were not included in the BP. As a result, over the next 80 years many formularies and pharmacopoeias were produced to fulfil this need.

A new need arose following the introduction of the National Health Insurance Act, which was passed by the Liberal Government in 1911, led by David Lloyd George. This established a scheme for the medical care of all employed workers, and could be described as the acorn from which the National Health Service oak tree grew. General practitioners were paid seven shillings a year for each patient on their panel, one shilling of which was meant to cover the costs of medicines. In the days before the NHI Act, most doctors, if they did not compound medicines themselves, had arrangements with a pharmacist who would be familiar with the complicated and elaborate mixtures which the doctors would prescribe. Not surprisingly small formularies, containing a selection of simple medicaments, were produced for NHI doctors in various neighbourhoods by the Local Panel Committees which represented the NHI doctors. A typical example of such an early NHI formulary would contain just 30 or so preparations, with all the titles expressed in Latin.

The number of these local formularies increased after the 1914–18 war. Often similar prescriptions had different titles in different formularies and sometimes the same title might have different ingredients in different formularies. Therefore, to reduce confusion, a number of local panel committees combined and produced formularies for larger areas.

In 1927, the BMA and the Retail Pharmacists Union took the lead and compiled a national formulary to serve NHI doctors throughout the United Kingdom. The first *National Health Insurance Formulary* was the result, published in 1929. It was a small book of 79 pages, containing 295 monographs, preceded by 'notes for guidance of medical practitioners in prescribing'. Even today these notes are topical, giving advice on the amounts which should be prescribed, the frequency of prescribing, and the need to be economically responsible.

The NHI Scheme did not cover hospital medical services, but from the beginning of the century most of the larger hospitals throughout the UK had their own published formularies; the medical staff would usually be restricted to prescribing those preparations in the formulary both for in-patients and for out-patients, but many of the visiting consultant staff had their own special concoctions which were not in any formulary.

Prescribing and dispensing policies remained much the same until the advent of the Second World War.

The National War Formulary

The conditions existing during the war made it imperative to exercise the strictest economy in prescribing. Even if the medicines themselves were readily available, their packing and distribution, often under difficult conditions, made demands on materials, manpower, and transport which could be justified only if the medicines were essential.

In January 1941, the Minister for Health appointed a small committee to prepare a National War Formulary (NWF). The formulary contained 'a selection of medicaments sufficient in range to meet the ordinary requirements for therapeutics'. It was for the use of all doctors whether working in general practice, in the community or in the hospital service. It listed 326 preparations, again the titles being in Latin; the doses were in the apothecaries' system.

British National Formulary

In 1948 the National Health Service (NHS) was created. This brought into one organisation GPs, the hospital services and the public health services. Continuing the publication of a *National Formulary*, for use throughout the NHS, was a matter for the B.M.A. and the Pharmaceutical Society, the two non-Governmental bodies which had been most closely concerned with the production of the NWF. These two bodies appointed a Joint Formulary Committee of 38 members to produce the *British National Formulary* (BNF). New editions of the BNF were produced about every three years from 1949 to 1976. Although some changes took place over those years, these were relatively few and slow to introduce.

Eventually, however, English replaced Latin and the metric system replaced the apothecaries' system. Slowly, the number of tonics and mixtures was reduced and new medicines, including the penicillins, tetracyclines, and corticosteriods were included. However, the tradition remained that the BNF, like the NWF, and the older NHI Formularies, was a selection of medicines. It was this 'selection' which eventually led to the BNF being less useful and acceptable to doctors. It did not reflect the advances being made by the pharmaceutical industry, and eventually it was perceived by doctors as being an 'irrelevance'.

The pharmaceutical industry capitalised on this, given that it had developed so many new and effective medicines, and developed competitive marketing techniques. The *Monthly Index of Medical Specialities* (MIMS) was introduced by an independent publishing company and the BNF, produced every three years, fell out of favour. It was estimated in 1976 that, of all doctors choosing to seek information on medicines, 80% of them referred to MIMS compared to 20% referring to the BNF. This led to a demand for a new type of *British National Formulary*, and eventually the Medicines Commission, concerned that doctors were not being advised from an authoritative and independent source, suggested a new and more comprehensive format.

It was decided that the old style BNF should be replaced by one which would be much more practical and useful for prescribing doctors. Initially, it was suggested that the Medicines Commission itself might become responsible for publishing the new BNF, but neither the BMA nor the Pharmaceutical Society were willing to hand over the copyright of the title to another body. Thus it was that the 'new' BNF remained the joint responsibility of these two professional bodies, and Colin Hitchings describes the current format and production of the BNF in detail in the next chapter.

The Limited List 'Formulary'

In November, 1984, the Government announced its controversial Limited List proposals which subsequently came into effect on 1 April 1985. This concept covered seven therapeutic areas and it was originally proposed that a formulary of just 31 products within these areas would meet 'all the clinical needs' of NHS patients.

Following strenuous public opposition to the proposals from the British Medical Association, other medical organisations and the Association of the British Pharmaceutical Industry, the Government increased the 'White List' of medicines that would remain available to NHS patients from the original 31 to 129. Subsequently the number increased to 154 as a result of reviews by the NHS Drugs Advisory Committee which was specifically set up to monitor the list.

The Government claimed at the time that the Limited List initiative would save the National Health Service at least £75 million each year, but during the Second Reading debate on the National Health Service and Community Care Bill in the House of Commons on December 11, 1989, a Conservative MP, Mr Michael Morris, asserted that the Government claims over savings achieved by the Limited List were 'as yet unsubstantiated'.

It is clear, however, that industry claims that the Limited List would inhibit research and development in the therapeutic areas covered were well justified. No new product licences have been issued in the respect of *innovative* medicines in these therapeutic categories since the introduction of the list in April 1985.

The increase in the number of products available to NHS patients (see Table 12.1) has been due entirely to previously 'black-listed' products being re-instated to the 'White List', as result of representations made to the NHS Drugs Advisory Committee.

The choice of medicines available for doctors to prescribe for NHS patients in these therapeutic areas has, therefore, not been widened or improved at all by the introduction of new or better medicines. In contrast, across the rest of the therapeutic spectrum, 70 new innovative medicines have been made available to NHS patients since 1985.

TABLE 12.1:   Products on the limited list 'White List' (i.e. prescribable for NHS patients)

	Nov 84	Feb 85	Nov 89
Antacids	5	16	27
Laxatives	2	23	21
Coughs and colds	7	18	22
Analgesics	5	24	34
Vitamins	8	34	37
Tonics/bitters	1	2	1
Benzodiazepines	3	12	12
Total	31	129	154

National Health Service Reforms

Leaping forward in time to the present day, much is still talked and written about formularies. Not surprisingly, the *Improving Prescribing* working papers[1] stimulated further discussion as to whether formularies should be encouraged and developed at various levels. However, in terms of a definitive list of what is available, it must be remembered that a formulary is defined as a *collection* of formulae or set forms, and that there is nothing in the definition about a limited or restricted collection. Seasoned collectors know that the best collections are those which are the most complete within their given spheres; a restricted collection frustrates by its incompleteness. It follows that formularies, to be maximally useful, and minimally frustrating, should be as complete as possible. The *British National Formulary* is a good and reasonably comprehensive example.

In spite of this argument, and the experiences learned with the 'limited list', the concept of local, limited or selective, formularies has been proposed, and at least one FHSA has produced its own version.[2] Although this idea might have its attractions for administrators and finance directors, arbitrary restriction of the choice of medicines available for doctors to be able to prescribe for patients is unacceptable, and Government Health Ministers have gone to great lengths to explain that selective formularies should not be binding on GPs and that they should be planned at practice level rather than being generated by regional or district committees.[3,4] This is now accepted throughout the primary health care service, as is reflected in the comments of several other contributors to this book.

Practice Formularies

What is now generally accepted is the educational value of devising a formulary at practice level, as this provides a strong intellectual stimulus for the doctors within the practice to think seriously about their patterns of prescribing. Professor Philip Reilly describes in detail the steps to be taken in, and the valuable experience which is gained by, drafting such a formulary in the last chapter in this book.

Several doctors who have experience in the use of practice formularies have written about them. For example, Beardon *et al.* have written about a formulary comprising 249 preparations of 132 medicines and medicine combinations which was prepared by the partners in a three doctor general practice in Scotland serving about 5,000 patients.[5] No attempt was made to change to generic prescribing nor were repeat prescription drugs altered. Introduction of the formulary in September 1981 was followed by an increase in the proportion of prescriptions containing drugs from the formulary from about 55% to more than 60% for both repeat and non-repeat prescriptions. The proportion of formulary drugs on non-repeat prescription reached a maximum of 78% within the first year with the additional influence of information feedback. Over the first year the level of formulary drugs used for both repeat and non-repeat prescribing levelled off to about 62%.

Even with these modest changes, when compared with the costs of general practice prescribing in Scotland as a whole, the introduction of the formulary resulted in savings of approximately 10% within the practice for the main ingredient costs both per patient and per prescription. Nevertheless, the practice doctors still had freedom to prescribe outside the formulary, the success of the formulary being that it generated a flexible prescribing policy, agreed by concensus amongst the prescribers concerned, allowances being made for non-formulary drugs to be used whenever the need arose.

Another paper describes how a survey of oral antibiotic prescriptions was carried out in a semi urban general practice.[6] From this a practice formulary was devised. The formulary was put into action and the results of its introduction reviewed after 12 months. There was a reduction in antibiotic costs, without an increase in the number of patient consultations, home visits or referral to hospital.

The production of the antibiotic formulary followed a business meeting of the nine doctor practice (in 1986) when the authors were appointed to produce a practice formulary. It was decided to carry out an initial audit of the current antibiotic prescribing, and this section was devised first. The current antibiotic prescribing patterns were noted, a literature search was conducted, and help was given from the North West Regional Drug Information Unit to devise the basic antibiotic formulary. The exercise included the submission of the draft formulary to all the members of the practice, the local pharmacists and the microbiologist for scrutiny and comment. It was introduced in 1986 and its effects assessed in February 1987.

Two further examples of the use of practice formularies are also of interest. An article by Grant *et al.* refers to a diverse group of general practitioners from separate practices who, over a period of one year, constructed a limited formulary for general practice use.[7] The formulary contained only 137 drugs and was intended to provide adequate and appropriate treatment for 90% of general practice patients. The authors concluded that the study provided a model for the development of agreed local formularies which do not infringe clinical freedom and offer an alternative to imposed limited lists as a means of reducing the costs of prescriptions. They found the development of such a list to have been an enjoyable and dynamic educational exercise.

It has been noted previously that compliance with a formulary is dependent on active involvement of the prescribing doctors in drafting it. Imposition of a formulary by whatever means arouses fears about clinical freedom. By aiming for only 90% compliance, the doctor is free to prescribe outside the formulary for those patients who have unusual conditions or for those who have not responded to the drugs within the formulary. While one doctor may achieve 100% compliance with a limited formulary, it is unlikely that doctors even from the same practice, let alone from separate practices, could do so.

The final example describes how, with the help of a research staff pharmacist, a voluntary preferred prescribing list, otherwise known as a general practice formulary, analogous to those already in use in some hospitals, was created, implemented and monitored within a group of five GPs and their trainees.[8] Cooperation between a pharmacist with knowledge of drug information, access to specialist advice and backup in the form of evaluated information from drug information centres, and the general practitioners was a key part of the exercise.

The formulary was well accepted with between 68.2% and 89.6% compliance in therapeutic classes corresponding to the 'limited list'. This method, the authors commented, enhanced the critical appraisal of prescribing rationale, took into the account the needs of doctors and patients and reduced costs. Such work highlights the value and scope of inter-disciplinary liaison between pharmacists, general practioners and clinical pharmacologists, and those involved believe it could prove beneficial on a national scale.

It was calculated that prescribing costs for the therapeutic groups were reduced by amounts ranging from 7.7% to 56.3%, amounting to an overall saving of 18.1% per year. The weight of evidence will, it is stated, clearly change with time and far from leaving the general practitioner with an outdated therapeutic armoury, the formulary approach enables the prescriber to update prescribing policies in the light of new evidence.

All the above examples – and indeed this chapter – refer to practice formularies. It almost goes without saying that the situation regarding hospital formularies is quite different. Firstly, the range of medicines needed in hospitals is very much smaller than that used in general practice; secondly, certain hospital medicines are not suitable for general practice use; and thirdly purchasing agreements may well influence the source of the medicines chosen for inclusion in the hospital formulary. Nevertheless, certain important principles are common to both hospital and practice based formularies: these include the need for constant review of the contents of the formulary, to ensure that it most cost-effectively meets the needs of patients, and that it reflects current medical opinion. Feely and his colleagues point out from their experience in Dublin[9] that continuous intervention, review, and feedback are required if a hospital – and presumably any other – formulary is to continue to fulfil those principles.

Conclusions

The Indicative Prescribing Scheme Working Paper emphasises that the development of a formulary is a time consuming task, though the educational value of drafting a practice formulary has been confirmed.

The arguments for including individual examples of medicines in given therapeutic groups in an inflexible limited formulary at any level – as opposed to providing the information about the complete range of available products, as is provided in the *British National Formulary* – are difficult to sustain, and that is now probably accepted throughout the United Kingdom. So long as costs are much of a muchness for equally effective medicines, or a more expensive medicine is recognised as being more effective, meaning that doctors may prescribe cost effectively what their patients need, there is no economic argument for producing a restricted formulary.

What is possibly not appreciated by prescribers well enough is need for the international pharmaceutical industry to maintain confidence in a research and development programme for the United Kingdom. Each company requires an income from each of its products, and so long as a company has a small share of a large market, it is more likely to survive than if it has no share at all in that market – just because the opportunity for choice has been arbitrarily reduced or eliminated.

Learning about medicines is important, and learning about their cost-effectiveness is an equally important part of responsible prescribing. If a practice so chooses, it can have a practice formulary, but the maintenance of that formulary must be a dynamic procedure. To assist that procedure, it is essential that doctors are provided with accurate and comprehensive information about the wide range of medicines available, from which at all times they must be free to choose.

References

1. *Improving Prescribing* (1990). Department of Health Working Papers. London, HMSO.
2. *General Practice Formulary.* (1990). Surrey Family Health Services Authority. Surbiton.
3. *Formularies for Prescribing.* Clarke, K. Speech in London, 16 February 1990.
4. Do I have to follow a formulary for prescribing? *Improving Prescribing* 1990; Para. 13.1. London, HMSO.
5. Beardon, P. H, Brown, S. V., Mowat, D. A., Grant, S. A. and McDevitt, D. G. (1987). Introducing a general formulary to drug practice – effects on practice prescribing costs. *Journal of the Royal College of General Practitioners* **37**, 305–307.
6. Needham, A., Brown, M. and Freeborn, F. (1988). Introduction and audit of a general practice antibiotic formulary. *Journal of the Royal College of Practitioners* **38**, 166–167.
7. Grant, G. B., Gregory, D. A. and van Zwanenberg, T. D. (1985). Development of a limited formulary for general practice. *Lancet* **i**, 1030–1032.
8. Green, P. E. (1985). The general practice formulary – its role in national therapeutics. *Journal of the Royal College of General Practitioners* **35**, 570–572.
9. Feely, J., Chan, R., Cocoman, L., Mulpeter, K. and O'Connor, P. (1990). Hospital formularies: need for continuous intervention. *British Medical Journal* **300**, 28–30.

13   The British National Formulary

Colin Hitchings

The British National Formulary, commonly known as the BNF, is a joint publication of the British Medical Association and the Royal Pharmaceutical Society of Great Britain. It was first produced in its current format in 1981 but the original BNF traces its history back to the 1930s. As the name implies, the original publication was indeed a national formulary and had its roots in the health insurance formularies of the 1930s. The various formularies then available were amalgamated following the outbreak of the Second World War and were united into a 'National War Formulary'. This provided a formulary incorporating substitutes for various drug materials which were in scarce supply due to the war situation.

The first BNF as such was produced in 1949 following the establishment of the National Health Service. The BNF was then published every two to three years and was highly selective in its format. The last of the original style BNFs covered the period of 1976 to 1978. By this time, the style of the BNF was rapidly becoming outdated and a need for a far more comprehensive formulary was established. It was determined that a much wider range of preparations should be covered and that more informed advice on the relative merits of preparations should be given. Although the title has been retained in the new format, the BNF in fact no longer contains a formulary for dispensing preparations. The new BNF is an objective and independent publication and is an up-to-date pocket book for rapid reference by both physicians and pharmacists and as such encourages rational and cost-effective prescribing.

The BNF is plainly visible throughout all hospitals and GP surgeries. The bright colour of each successive edition is readily visible and the often dog-eared copies give evidence of the usefulness and frequency of use! Nurses and other health care professionals use the BNF regularly as an educational tool as do both medical and pharmacy under-graduates.

A Dental Practitioners Formulary is incorporated within the BNF every two years and contains advice on the specialised requirements of products for dentistry.

The BNF is distributed by the Department of Health every six months to all doctors and pharmacists in the NHS and to all hospital wards and departments in the NHS. Similarly, every two years the joint Dental Practitioners' Formulary and BNF is distributed to all dentists in the NHS. Medical and pharmacy students also receive copies periodically. Approximately 160,000 copies of each edition are printed.

Examination of the first edition of the new BNF published in 1981 indicates how radical the revision was at that time. The title headings of the various sections also indicate that the format adopted would appear to have been largely successful as the main headings have been little altered over the ten years of publication. The first edition consisted of the following main sections:

Guidance on Prescribing

General Information;
Prescription Writing;
Prescribing for Children;
Prescribing for the Elderly;
Prescribing in Liver Disease;
Prescribing in Renal Impairment;
Adverse Reactions to Drugs;
Controlled Drugs and Drug Dependence.

Emergency Treatment of Poisoning

Classified Notes on Drugs and Preparations

1. Gastro-intestinal System;
2. Cardiovascular System;
3. Respiratory System;
4. Central Nervous System;
5. Infections;
6. Endocrine System;
7. Obstetrics and Gynaecology;
8. Malignant Disease and Immunosuppression;
9. Nutrition and Blood;
10. Musculoskeletal and Joint Diseases;
11. Eye;
12. Ear, Nose and Oropharynx;
13. Skin;
14. Immunological Products and Vaccines;
15. Anaesthesia;
Appendix 1: Drug Interactions;
Appendix 2: Intravenous Additives;
Appendix 3: Borderline Substances;
Formulary;
Dental Practitioners' Formulary;
Index to Manufacturers.

Each main chapter is introduced with a page or two of general information relating to the particular subject and pertinent matters.

The various sub-groups are then addressed and again general advice and comment provided on each sub-group. The individual monographs then follow in each sub-group, each monograph consisting of:

Indications;
Cautions;
Contra-indications;
Side Effects;
Dose – by various routes both adult and child if appropriate.

Each proprietary preparation is then listed, the form in which it is available, the quantity of active ingredient and the basic cost as used in pricing prescriptions. Additional information is provided where it is thought relevant – for example, diluents are indicated in the entries for certain creams and ointments where lower strengths may be prescribed.

The classification system can best be demonstrated by example, using Chapter 5 : Infections:

5. *Infections*

    5.1. Antibacterial Drugs;
    5.2. Antifungal Drugs;
    5.3. Antiviral Drugs;
    5.4. Antiprotozoal Drugs;
    5.5. Anthelmintics.

Each of these five sub-groups is then divided further e.g. 5.5:

    5.5.1. Drugs for Threadworms;
    5.5.2. Ascaricides;
    5.5.3. Taenicides;
    5.5.4. Drugs for Hookworms;
    5.5.5. Schistosomicides;
    5.5.6. Filaricides;
    5.5.7. Drugs for Guinea Worms;
    5.5.8. Drugs for Strongyloidiasis.

Each of these further sub-divisions then contains the individual drug monographs.

On examining the current BNF some ten years later, the changes in format are minimal and reflect contemporary concerns and interests. The formulary section has now been deleted completely, its demise having been hardly noticed. The sections on Prescribing in Liver Disease and in Renal Impairment have been moved to separate appendices; a new section has been added on prescribing in terminal care and additional appendices have appeared on pregnancy, breast feeding and cautionary and advisory labels together with the inclusion of the CSM yellow cards for the reporting of adverse drug reactions.

Joint Formulary Committee

The Joint Formulary Committee is collectively responsible for the production on a six-monthly basis of the BNF. The Formulary Committee is kept small so as to allow the flexibility required for a six-monthly publication.

It is composed of three nominees from both the BMA and the RPSGB as joint owners of the title together with three nominees from the Department of Health representing the main purchaser of the book (Figure 13.1). The committee is serviced by joint secretaries, one from each of the two professional bodies.

Data for the BNF are gathered from numerous sources. Each section of the BNF has an expert adviser who is a practising clinician. The Joint Formulary Committee, whilst it is an independent body, heeds much of the official guidance that is available; for example, it closely follows the Department of Health Guidelines on Vaccines. Likewise, warnings issued by official bodies are introduced into the BNF. Data sheets are always studied in some detail but the BNF, on occasions, will take a different view. All main journals are monitored and if necessary expert advice sought on key issues.

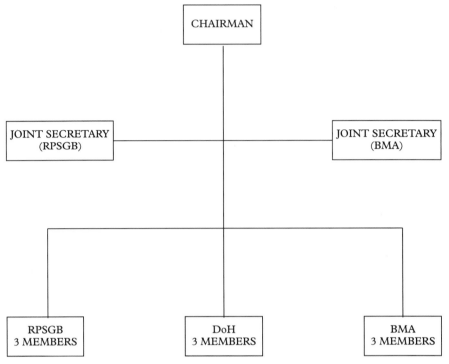

Figure 13.1:   The joint formulary committee.

Aims of the BNF

The overall aim of the BNF is to promote effective, safe and economical use of medicines. It is a feature of the BNF that it now includes all the prescription-only medicines which are on the UK market and many more besides. It is, therefore, a comprehensive document which provides independent comment on all the medicines covered. Smaller print size is often used for both medicines and preparations which, in the view of the Joint Formulary Committee, may not be as effective as alternative therapy. Likewise, an indication of the drug costs are included. Initially this was done by banding from letter A, costing up to 20p, through to letter G which was over £4.50. More recently, however, basic net prices have been introduced into the BNF in order to provide a better indication of relative costs. A unit of 20 is used as the basis for comparison excepting where suitable original packs are available and these are costed instead. The BNF prices are of course, only suitable for making comparisons and are not appropriate for direct costing to patients.

The Terms of Reference of the Joint Formulary Committee are:

1. to reflect the views of the respective organisations;

2. to decide changes in policy, format and publication frequency;

3. to appoint an Editorial Team.

The full committee meets twice for each BNF edition.

An Editorial Team headed by the Executive Editor is responsible for:

1. checking and confirming the BNF data and ensuring their correctness.
2. identifying problems and seeking the help of expert advisers.
3. processing feedback from the pharmaceutical industry, particularly that relating to data sheets.
4. co-ordinating fresh data generated for committee decisions, particularly in those areas that are controversial.
5. continuing the up-dating and routine printing of the BNF on a six-monthly basis.

The inter-relationship of those responsible for producing the BNF is shown diagrammatically in Figure 13.2.

BNF Classification System

The classification system which has been adopted by the BNF has become universally accepted and is used by many formularies and by various computer systems. The classification system has indeed been adopted by the Prescription Pricing Authority and is in universal use throughout the UK.

The Prescription Pricing Authority (PPA) is not only responsible for, as its name implies, the pricing of prescriptions, but also for the production of

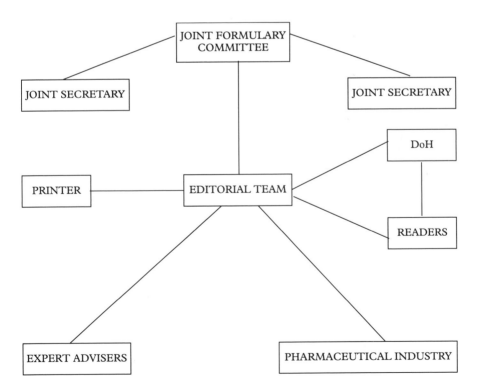

Figure 13.2: Inter-relationships of the joint formulary committee.

detailed information for general practitioners on their prescribing habits. Chapter 5 specifically covers the generation of prescribing data by the PPA. The system adopted for this procedure is the classification system developed by the Joint Formulary Committee for the BNF. Occasionally, of course, changes have to be made to the classification system but in view of the universal use of the BNF system, these are kept to a minimum. Any such changes are published in the front of each edition of the BNF.

Local Formularies

The production of local formularies in hospitals has been officially encouraged over many years. Such formularies exist in hospitals and districts throughout the length and breadth of the UK. The classification system adopted for these local formularies is again almost universally that developed by the BNF.

Until recently local formularies were almost entirely the domain of the hospital service but their influence on GP prescribing gradually became recognised. Patients attending hospital out-patient departments and in-patients on discharge would receive medication in accordance with that hospital's formulary. Unless there were very specific reasons for change the GP would usually continue the hospital initiated medication. The production of local formularies by and for GPs is now officially promulgated, particularly at practice level, and those that have been produced again mostly use the BNF classification.

BNF Monographs

The BNF continually monitors licensed indications for drugs and it therefore provides a useful guide to any changes introduced. Similarly, it monitors doses and indeed, on occasions, gives advice which reflects clinical practice and not necessarily data sheet information. It must, though, be recognised that only data sheets contain information which has been approved by the CSM. All dose changes are, incidentally, indicated again at the front of the BNF.

International Influences

The BNF has become an authoritative document throughout the English speaking world and is purchased worldwide. The format of the BNF has been virtually copied in a number of countries, indeed not just the English speaking world as Greece has adopted an almost identical format. It is said that 'Imitation is the greatest form of flattery'. Other countries around the world have also 'flattered' the BNF, from the Antipodes, to North America to Europe.

Conclusion

The British National Formulary, in its post 1980 format, is now firmly established in its current role and accepted as a most useful source document for all aspects of prescribing. It is produced every six months and as such is a dynamic production which continually keeps abreast of changes. This ability to adjust and adapt rapidly is one of the secrets of the success of the publication and whilst able to do this, it should continue its progressive role in influencing prescribing.

14 General Practice Formularies: Advice on Drafting and Practice Use

Philip Reilly

Definition

A General Practice Formulary (G.P.F.) is a voluntary preferred selection of medications assembled by the practice with or without the help of a variety of sources of some expertise. Several practices may be involved, working together to produce the selection of medications which they will usually prescribe. Other colleagues such as pharmacists and specialists, particularly pharmacologists, may also contribute.

The starting point must inevitably be from where the practice finds itself. PACT data (and the equivalent in Scotland and Northern Ireland) will clarify the practice position to a considerable extent, but not completely as will be seen later.

A General Practice Formulary may be based on the therapeutic classes as in the British National Formulary. Another format consists of the selection of medications on the basis of clinical conditions. Thus the cardiovascular section would include congestive heart failure, hypertension, and so on. This format, based on clinical conditions, is helpful for general practitioners who have to contend with conditions which can either be precisely defined (such as anaemia) or be quite non-specific (such as dizziness).

Underlying Assumptions

A General Practice Formulary is intended[1]

1. to provide simple, adequate and appropriate treatment for the vast majority of patients presenting with common conditions – *where the prescribing of a drug is thought necessary*;
2. to be useful and acceptable to a diverse group of general practitioners in a range of practice settings;
3. to encourage generic prescribing where this is appropriate;
4. to avoid the inclusion of any drug which has recently been introduced until there is evidence of its superiority over standard treatment. This will not result in patients being deprived of the newest and, by implication, the best medications. In fact there has been enough evidence over the past decade, in the withdrawal of new preparations because of unacceptable side effects in patients, to make general practitioners circumspect. In any case, critical scrutiny of new preparations by general practitioners who are involved in formulary construction is highly desirable for all concerned, including the patient and the pharmaceutical industry. In meeting innovations such doctors are likely to appreciate the value of particular new preparations;

121

5. to take into account the cost of drugs as an important but not paramount factor. In fact adequate treatment of, and medication for, some conditions (such as asthma) may well increase prescribing costs. It is essential that patients receive effective medication and that this is monitored through normal peak flow readings, plus appropriate referrals and an absence of emergency admission. If this situation pertains, overall costs to the NHS will be substantially reduced;

6. to exclude medications that are usually initiated in hospital care (for instance, most cytotoxics). However medications for common conditions recommended by hospital should be scrutinised as choice of preparation may not necessarily concur with formulary policy. The diplomatic, sensible and professional way of dealing with this is to ensure that the local hospital formulary contains *and marks* the preparations from the general practice formulary with an asterisk. Placed prominently at the front of the hospital formulary should be a statement such as 'drugs marked with an asterisk* have been selected for inclusion in the local general practice formularies and are therefore particularly suited for general practitioner prescribing when the patient has been discharged'.

7. to provide a useful tool for teaching and learning;

8. to be modified predominantly by general practitioners for general practitioners on a regular basis.

Why the Need for a Formulary?

So large is the volume of information and so great the range of preparation that the general practitioner is in danger of being overloaded. At least two dangers arise; firstly, general practitioners just respond to trends in their prescribing data without any thought of policy formation, or secondly, general practitioners may just habituate to much of the data fed back to them. The passive nature of this system, despite the presence of sanctions, may not lead to changes. Two further points come to mind – active involvement in any process is much more likely to lead to change and in any case prescribers have received substantial amounts of instruction in pharmacology and therapeutics. In other words how can prescribing, a central activity in any clinician's role, be maintained as an area of professional competence, even expertise?

Effective prescribing comprises several skills such as being able to assimilate or access relevant pharmacological and therapeutic information, to update knowledge, as well as to cope with new concepts. Being able to communicate with patients is very important – wants and needs are not the same and effective negotiation and education is always a part of doctor/patient relationships. Being able to maximise compliance is becoming even more essential as chronic diseases increase in prevalence. Finally, the ability to organise and manage a repeat prescribing system operationally and clinically is vital. Repeat prescribing is a significant and perhaps permanent feature of UK general practice.

Feedback of prescribing data alone, regardless of how sophisticated, is unlikely to enable general practitioners to become competent prescribers. In any case the situation is compounded by other realities. Firstly, in dealing with many common conditions the general practitioner is usually faced with a range of preparations from which to choose. Secondly, the range of choice, thanks in part to an innovative pharmaceutical industry, frequently changes. Inevitably therefore, general practitioners must adopt an additional strategy to cope effectively as prescribers. They must become active, make selections, and develop criteria that enable them to make good selections. Such activity is rigorous, voluntary, professionally satisfying, likely to maximise good patient care – it is called formulary construction. Cost containment is a likely but not inevitable byproduct though efficacy, safety and acceptability to patients should be in the vast majority of situations.[2]

How to go about Constructing a Formulary

There are three tasks involved where satisfactory answers must be found and sound policies developed.

1. *Developing Good Selection Criteria for Choosing Medications*

Why should prescribers select? General practitioners largely manage common illnesses. Prescribing for each of these illnesses usually offers a wide choice. At least 80% of patients in general practice with any given common illness will respond to an established medication. A small minority will require considerable therapeutic effort in effecting a cure, improvement or maintenance. Selection together with some flexibility is therefore inevitable. Provided this '80/20' rule is observed, cost containment is rarely a major issue because cost effectiveness is being addressed. The majority (80% approx) of patients in receiving established medications are, by definition, cost effective (though this does not mean that further improvement is not possible). Neither does it mean that the majority (80%) are getting cheap second rate medications. In dealing with the minority (20%) of patients not responding to established medications, the prescriber can be appropriately radical, outside the formulary selection. Formularies in general practice should imply flexibility.

The challenge for the prescriber is therefore to identify to which group the patient with common illness belongs – the 80% majority or the 20% minority – and to prescribe accordingly. Such a professional approach from the prescriber should also mean that patients get the medications appropriate to their clinical condition.

How therefore are medications selected for a practice formulary? It is relatively easy to think of characteristics a drug must possess. Effective, safe, economic, appropriate to the patient's condition as well as acceptable, are all desirable characteristics. It is however quite a challenge to operationalise these features in such a way that a choice can be made between the various preparations in a given therapeutic class. A simple, though at times difficult exercise, consists in itemising specific selection criteria, as shown in Figure 1.

Selection criteria may vary in certain therapeutic classes and should be extended as much as possible so that the best choices can be made. Therapeutic classes such as non-steroidal anti-inflammatory drugs, where there are many medications, involve one sort of selection process. Choice of preparations which lower lipid levels, where there are relatively few preparations as yet, involve a different process. These processes of selection vary with almost every therapeutic class.

Specific selection criteria*	Names of various medications				
	Drug A	Drug B	Drug C	Drug D	etc
Aim (in use)					
Observations					
Alternatives					
Duration of course					
Metabolism					
Interactions					
Route + dosage					
Unwanted effects					
Cost					

The names of medications are placed across the top of the sheet. The criteria are listed on the left hand side of the page. These criteria put pertinent questions to the selectors who may include other disciplines (pharmacists, pharmacologists etc) as well as *all* the practice doctors. The drugs chosen have the most acceptable profile.

Definitions of Specific Selection Criteria*

Aim: what is the aim/purpose in using the proposed medication?

Observations: what observations have to be made when using the proposed medications?

Alternatives: what are the alternatives (medication and otherwise) available?

Duration :   how long does the medication have to be taken?

Metabolism: how does the body handle the medication?

Interactions: what interactions (anticipated and others) might be observed?

Route + Dosage: self explanatory

Unwanted effects: what are these and how acceptable?

Figure 14.1

Many relevant prescribing issues are raised though not all can be settled. In any case the selection process is ongoing and is really a major learning opportunity in which doctors build up a structured approach to selection which has a wide application for established as well as new medications.

2. *Will the Group (GPs and Others) Work Cohesively and Effectively Together to Produce Prescribing Policies?*

When practices are observed examining their own prescribing data, they (as a group) progress or fail to progress through a series of stages.[3]

(a) *Defensive* comments: e.g. 'we are not very good at this' etc.;
(b) *Projective* comments: e.g. 'we are the sort of practice which . . .';

(c) *Deficiency Acknowledged*: this is especially seen when the group has its own data in front of it;

(d) *Dialogue*: this is particularly noted when everybody knows each others' data;

(e) *Agreement/Disagreement*: how productive this exchange is really depends on how the practice group handles the range of committed and other views;

(f) *Policy Development*: the practice group needs some form of working consensus as well as good sources of information so that members can address and complete a series of tasks;

(g) *Implement Change*: such change must be carried out efficiently and in a committed manner;

(h) *Check that Change has Taken Place*: practice organisation is needed here as well as commitment.

Practice groups will not progress beyond the stage of agreement/disagreement unless they work together regularly (monthly) and in a manner that caters for the needs of the group/practice members as well as the task in hand.

It is important to ensure that as many as possible of the practice group actually do the work of setting criteria and applying them. Some of the group could later challenge the validity of the chosen criteria when, for example, the data show an unacceptable level of compliance. In attempting to generate a feeling of responsibility for the criteria chosen, the practice group enlarges and lengthens them. Such developments result in criteria that are less precise and usually less easily audited. Precise criteria are essential if data are to be used and not left unconsidered – the so-called 'orphan' data.[4] Participants in audit respond best to specific items which, if not attained, are remedied by an education programme that is focused, personal and occurs soon after the audit exercise has stopped. Success is most likely when involvement has been active, addressing issues documented by clinical research and selected for its importance to patients' well-being and for correctability by doctor performance.

The management of change and the development of innovation are demanding. The practice group needs to know when change is really necessary. The whole process must seem and actually be possible. The impression and the reality will be more successful if the whole process is shared by all the participants. Both practice and individual practitioner identity must be reinforced.

3. *How Will the Practice/Group Handle Operational Problems such as Repeat Prescribing?*

A repeat prescribing system, adequately policed, is not just acceptable but very necessary in current UK general practice. Good information systems allow repeat prescriptions to be printed by a computer with policy decisions built in, thus saving valuable time. However the initial impact of formulary construction could be significant.

The practice will wish to consider policies as applied to patients receiving repeat prescriptions. In the light of any changes, will any or all such patients have to be seen? What explanation will be given? How can the practice ensure that such explanations will be understood? At least one third, and in some cases up to half, of all doctor-patient contacts face to face (direct) or otherwise (indirect) are through the repeat prescribing system. The practice will have to explain change, systematically and in an acceptable way, to various categories of patients, including the elderly, the housebound, and so on. Such changes will have to be clinically indicated, as safe as possible, understood and complied with willingly, and in as informed a manner as possible.

How to Maintain a Practice Formulary

Successful initial construction of a general practice formulary involves multidisciplinary activity as described above. Use and acceptance of the formulary is strongly related to a wide network of actively participating general practitioners. Such ownership can be fostered and strengthened by the formation of User Groups.

These groups are essentially self-directed though they will agree to monitor a particular section of the formulary and update it as required. They can be resourced with substantial prescribing information about the particular area/therapeutic class they wish to develop. Apart from information, ordinary pharmacists plus drug information pharmacists can supply relevant data. This can be added to the detailed feedback already available through PACT. Other professionals can be involved, including pharmacologists, though pharmacists are the other most common professionals.

User groups could well become a useful forum for exchange of ideas which can be collated centrally. Examples of such exchanges include:

(1) the development of cost-benefit analyses which may well enable the best type of choices of medication to be made;

(2) access of a 'rep' from the pharmaceutical industry. This might well represent a useful opportunity for particular companies. Occasionally, sound post-marketing surveillance studies could be carried out;

(3) studies which could effectively examine issues of variation in prescribing between areas which seem similar – does such variation represent over or under treatment?

(4) continuing exploration of factors (for example, age structure or specific morbidity) which may well effect the indicative prescribing amounts now being set.

At the same time, participating practices will feel that they are involved and making an effective and essential contribution to maintaining a practice formulary.

Conclusion

Given the range of skills (see above) required to be a competent prescriber two strategies are essential. The production of sophisticated feedback (PACT etc) even reinforced by financial sanction is actually not enough. The second strategy of formulary construction implying active involvement, but nevertheless voluntary in nature, represents the sort of educational, collaborative and professional activity essential for competence in prescribing. It is not a cost containment exercise bent on giving the patient less than optimal medication.

It is not an activity inimical to the pharmaceutical industry. It represents general practitioners reclaiming fundamental areas of competence and in a manner that will sustain them through their professional careers.

References

1. Grant, G. B., Gregory, D. A., van Zwanenberg, T. D. (1985). Development of a limited formulary for general practice. *Lancet*, 1030–31.
2. Beardon, P. H. G., Brown, S. V., Mowat, D. A. E., Grant, J. A. and McDevitt, D. G. (1987). Introducing a drug formulary to general practice – effects on practice prescribing costs. *Journal of the Royal College of General Practitioners* 37, 305–307.
3. Reilly, P. M. (1985). An Audit of Prescribing by Peer Review. *MD Thesis. Queen's University, Belfast.*
4. Nelson, A. R. (1976). Orphan Data and the closed loop. *New England Journal of Medicine* 295, 617–619.
5. Green, P. E. (1985). The General Practice Formulary – its role in rational therapeutics. *Journal of the Royal College of General Practitioners* 35, 570–572.

15 Responsible Prescribing: The Hospital Community Interface

Michael Orme

Responsible prescribing of medicines should mean that medicines are prescribed and used in such a way that the maximum clinical benefit is obtained from them at the lowest possible cost. This does not mean that the cost of a medicine is the most important fact to consider when prescribing since our aim must be to produce the maximum therapeutic benefit that we can. In the past the cost of medicines was rarely considered and most doctors, until recently, probably had little idea of the cost of the medicines they prescribed. The advent of PACT (see Chapters 3 and 4) has changed that fundamentally and it is interesting to see that many general practitioners have responded to data about their own prescribing in a very positive manner. Unfortunately, prescribers in hospital do not yet have the sort of information available in the community and will probably need to wait for a few years to receive comprehensive data. The cost of medicines is important since this is rising steadily and some medicines are very expensive. The medicines bill for the NHS is currently about £2000 million per year and represents the biggest single expenditure item apart from salaries. Medicines are expensive because of the time and effort that goes into their development. In order to produce a medicine that is as effective and safe as possible it will now take up to 15 years, at a cost of up to £100 million, to develop a new chemical entity. Virtually all new medicines are produced as a result of research in the pharmaceutical industry and clearly they need to recoup their development costs. Since the effective patent life has been steadily eroded the time available to regain those costs has been slowly lessening. It is therefore encouraging to hear of plans in the EEC to extend the patent life of proprietary medicines throughout Europe.

The cost of individual medicines can be exemplified by centoxin – a new monoclonal IgM antibody (HA–1A) which binds specifically to the lipid A domain of endotoxin produced by gram negative bacteria. Centoxin has been shown to be clinically effective in the treatment of severe gram negative septicaemia with a reduction in mortality from 49% to 30%.[1] However, although the treatment with centoxin only requires a single dose, that dose costs £2200. Other medicines which have recently been given product licences are also expensive. Tissue plasminogen activator (tPA) which is useful in the thrombolytic treatment of coronary artery occlusion (myocardial infarct) costs about £800 per dose in the United Kingdom although the cost is greater in some other countries. Recent studies, however, have shown that streptokinase has a very similar efficacy and side effect profile and since it costs about ten times less than tPA in most British and many European centres, streptokinase is usually preferred. However in the USA, where drug cost is at present less of a problem, tPA is preferred. Clearly, guidelines for the use of these medicines are important but they are in essence hospital based medicines (although general practice trials of thrombolytic therapy are in progress). In other cases expensive medicines are used in both the hospital and in the community. Thus octreotide, recently marketed for patients with the carcinoid syndrome, costs £950 to the NHS if used at its highest recommended dose. Ondansetron may be better than other antiemetics in some patients receiving cancer chemotherapy yet its cost is currently imposing limitations on its use, mainly in hospitals. Erythropoetin, which markedly improves the quality of life of patients with chronic renal disease, is not used to its optimum because of the costs of the medicine – either in hospital or in the community.[2]

However, the cost of a medicine should not be the sole arbiter of its use in clinical situations. Sometimes the use of an expensive drug will allow a patient to spend less time in hospital or save costs in other ways. Thus the use of isotretinoin (although expensive at up to £350 for a four month course) actually reduces the total costs of treating patients with acne over a five year period[3] as well as being more efficacious than other therapy. Expensive medicines may also allow patients to return to productive work more quickly and in the past we have not been good at looking at comparative costings that come out of different pockets. Thus a medicine like sumatriptan although expensive at £40 per injection might well be justified if it allowed a patient with migraine to return to work rapidly. Research needs to be done on this sort of area and it is to be hoped that the new Research and Development Committee of the NHS will encourage this sort of service research. In other cases medicines that do not yet have a product licence may be very expensive and this will primarily occur in hospital. Thus I was called in by the Managers of Christie Hospital in Manchester to advise following an outcry over the use of interleukin 2. A patient with renal cell carcinoma had been denied therapy with interleukin 2 partly on cost grounds and partly because the efficacy of interleukin 2 in this situation was not good.[4] The recent change of SIFT (Supplementary Income for Teaching) to include research and so to become SIFTR gives a possible route for funding this type of activity since clearly the medicine in this situation is being used in a research setting.

We can thus expect new medicines to be more and more expensive as time goes on and recent changes in the NHS have made managers look ever more closely at the costs of the treatment provided in the NHS. This applies to both hospitals and the community. Since the formation of many NHS Trusts on April 1 1991, hospitals are becoming more cost conscious and at the same time general practitioners have either become fundholders with an actual drug budget, or have been given indicative prescribing amounts. This will increase with another wave of new NHS Trusts and fundholding practices in April 1992. Thus financial pressures will build up both in hospitals and in the community. Hospitals have been under pressure to save costs on medicines over the last 10 years or more. The drug budget has been seen as one of the easier ways of saving money in hospital since it is hard to save on salaries. Thus most hospitals now have their own formularies and these have certainly helped to contain costs.[5] However, the continued pressures on the budget have led to costs being offloaded onto the community and it is this area that is particularly problematical.

Prescribing is essentially a community activity with 80% of prescribing being carried out by general practitioners. Thus in my own region (Mersey Region) the total budget for medicines is £120 million of which only about £20 million is prescribed by and dispensed in hospitals. The cost of dispensing medicines is essentially greater in the community partly because the medicines themselves are more expensive since discounts are less easily obtainable. In addition, the dispensing charge is slightly higher overall in the community. This is largely offset by VAT differences. Hospitals have to pay VAT (currently 17.5%) on the medicines they dispense but in the community medicines are exempt from VAT. The reasoning behind this anomaly is unclear and the Department of Health is said to have formed a working party to try to resolve the issue. I fear it is the nature of government that the issue will be regularised by charging VAT on medicines dispensed in the community. One of the good things to emerge from the latest NHS changes is the chance that it gives us to bring together hospital and community activity. The government publication 'Improving Prescribing' (Working Paper No. 2 of working for patients)[6] tells us to bring together hospital and community prescribing. Regional Health Authorities are now responsible for both hospital activities and community activities (the latter through the Family Health Service Authorities (FHSAs), the successors to the FPC). The aim is to combine the two drug budgets by April 1992 and if we are able to look at the whole regional drug budget as a single entity, considerable rationalisation could occur. However it is apparent that at present the hospital drug budget is cash limited while the community drug budget is not. General practitioners have been reassured by the Secretary of State for Health that they will be able to prescribe the medicines their patients need, regardless of cost. This reassurance is seen somewhat sceptically by many general practitioners because of the actual drug budget (for fund holders) or the indicative prescribing amount of which they have been notified. We will return to this issue later.

Issues at the Interface

There are a number of issues at the hospital community interface which are currently causing problems and their resolution is not likely to be in the immediate future.

1. *Communication*

I regard this as a central issue at the interface and it is clearly a two way process. Not only do hospitals communicate badly with general practitioners but the process is true in reverse. In the interests of overall economies, secretarial services are often reduced in hospital and it is not unusual for a discharge summary or an outpatient letter to take six weeks to reach the GP after the patient has been last seen in hospital. On discharge from the ward it is regular practice to send a brief handwritten note to the GP which describes the medication prescribed on discharge. Often however these letters are illegible and it is the typed discharge summary that is important. As a result the GP (or the receptionist) has to waste time telephoning the hospital to find out which medicines the patient is supposed to be taking. If the system is to work well we must improve our methods of communicating. Hospital discharge summaries must be completed sooner and much greater use of the FAX machinery should avoid delays inherent in the postal service.

2. *Formularies*

The production of local hospital formularies should be encouraged but I see no need for a regional formulary since the British National Formulary provides what a regional formulary would give. There are differences between each hospital formulary and this variation allows the pharmaceutical industry at least some hope of an open market. Many general practitioners are also producing their own formularies and this shows a healthy interest in their own prescribing activities. Many hospital formularies cover only inpatient activities but whether the formularies are expanded to cover outpatient activities or not, formulary designers need to look more closely at the needs of the local general practitioners. Thus there should be general practitioner representation on hospital formulary committees and revision of the formulary should involve consultation with the local GPs. This can perhaps be best done through the FHSAs with the medical and pharmaceutical advisers playing a lead role.

(a) *Generic Prescribing*

This topic is covered in full elsewhere in the book (see chapter 8) but a few comments are relevant here to the formulary situation. Generic prescribing is slowly becoming more popular. It is regular practice in hospitals, and in the community about 40% of prescriptions are written generically. The advantages of generic prescribing to me outweigh the disadvantages. One of the claimed disadvantages is the quality of the product but this is mostly based on old data. In the past some generic medicines (eg digoxin) did have uneven bioavailability but this is not true today although we need to watch the parallel import situation. The biggest disadvantage to me of generic prescribing in the community is the situation that may arise at each new dispensing of a generic prescription. One month a patient, for example, on diphenylhydantoin (phenytoin) may be given red and white capsules but the following month may receive white tablets. The patient, if no explanation is given, will reasonably feel that his treatment has been changed and will complain to both pharmacist and GP. This will then take valuable time to reassure the patient but even so some patient confidence may be lost. If this situation could be improved I think generic prescribing would become more widespread. One way might be for generic formulations of any particular medicine to be standardised throughout a region, through a contract with a major generic pharmaceutical company. This is however more difficult than it sounds since extensive discussions would need to take place with the community pharmacists who are independent contractors in the system.

(b) *Loss Leaders*

Since hospital drug budgets are so tight from the cash point of view there is an inevitable tendency to accept a heavily discounted price regardless of the cost of the medicine in the community. The most obvious example of this occurred many years ago when the new benzodiazepines, diazepam and chlordiazepoxide were provided free to many hospitals. Marketing departments of pharmaceutical companies know that hospitals exert a great influence on the prescribing of local

GPs. A general practitioner will rarely change the prescription of a patient who has been recommended to have a particular medicine by the local hospital consultant. A current example is the drug Frumil® which is a combination of frusemide and amiloride. Frumil is heavily discounted to hospitals with the price in many cases being 25% of that in the community. The generic equivalent Co-amilofrus does not easily come to mind compared to the name Frumil®. Thus hospitals will buy Frumil and once the patient is discharged from hospital this product will continue to be prescribed. This is not a very efficient way to use NHS resources as a whole. In future, I feel that when hospital formularies are being revised we should pay attention to the cost of medicines in the community. Medicines will be chosen first and foremost for their therapeutic efficacy, but where two products are seen as therapeutically equivalent, the cost of the medicine in the community should be the main consideration rather than solely the discount price available in hospital.

Greater attention to the use of generic medicines in the community and to the loss leader situation will save a large amount of money which can be better used in the judicious use of the expensive medicines already discussed. Thus the cost of Frumil® in England and Wales in 1990 exceeded £20 million and I am convinced this money could have been better spent.

3. *Discharge Medications*

Most hospitals have been in the habit of prescribing and dispensing 14 days supply of medicines for patients on discharge from hospital. However, financial limitations have persuaded many of them to cut this supply to seven days. A study in South Derbyshire[7] showed that cutting the length of discharge treatment in this way would save £40,000 annually with a negligible effect on patient care. However the cost saved in hospital would have been more than offset by increased costs in the community. In addition, particularly in deprived inner city areas where communication is often poorer, the necessary information may not get to the GP. Thus many general practitioners objected to the increased workload involved at a time when they were already heavily committed. It seems to me that a 14 day supply of medicines is the correct length of treatment to provide when patients leave hospital but such a move would have cost implications for most hospitals.

4. *A and E Prescribing*

Patients attending the Accident and Emergency department of hospitals are often dispensed only two or three days supply of medicine unless the full course of therapy would need only four or five days treatment (eg some infections treated with antibiotics). In these cases a full course of therapy is given. On some occasions only giving two or three days supply of medicine causes problems for the GP and increased costs for the community. In general, however, surveys have shown that most patients treated in the A and E department do not need more than two or three days supply and to give a week's supply could be wasteful. Clearly, therefore, good communications are essential to and from the A and E department.

5. *Outpatient Prescribing*

It has long been established that 'the duty of prescribing for a particular element of a patient's treatment rests with the doctor who at the time has clinical responsibility for that element.' This has come from numerous directives from the Department of Health (eg HN (76) 69) and has been repeated over the years. However problems continue to arise. One of the main problems has been in deciding whether the hospital consultant or the general practitioner has clinical responsibility for any element of a patient's care. In theory a GP may refer a patient to a consultant for advice and treatment or for advice only. In any case the GP usually retains overall responsibility for a patient's care. There has been a definite trend to offload the prescribing costs of outpatient therapy onto the general practitioner and this applies to both regular outpatient care and to the use of complicated or expensive therapies. The concept of shared care is well known in some areas of medicine (eg obstetrics) and is beginning to come in some other areas (eg diabetes care) and these moves should be encouraged. If a patient is referred to hospital for advice on the treatment of, say, hypertension the responsibility for prescribing will need to be defined. It would seem reasonable in the initial period for the hospital to have responsibility when the patient attends the hospital say every two to eight weeks. However as the treatment is stabilized the hospital may wish to see the patient every six to 12 months for review or research purposes and at this stage it could be made clear that clinical responsibility is being returned to the GP. In the treatment of certain disease states (eg transplantation) or in the use of certain medicines (eg cytotoxic drugs, erythropoetin, sandostatin) the GP cannot be expected to have the detailed knowledge necessary to monitor the drug therapy effectively and in this situation the hospital specialist should retain clinical responsibility and with it the responsibility for prescribing. Again, good communication in these areas of care will be vital for success. If a hospital does prescribe and dispense medicines for a patient it would be sen-sible for four weeks treatment to be given rather than the current practice of a limit on two weeks supply. Again this will increase the costs on hospital budgets but save money in the community. Giving a month's supply rather than two weeks will also save on prescription charges for a patient where these need to be paid. It is to be hoped that if these policies were to be implemented they would be applied flexibly. In some cases, because of transport difficulties, it will be much more convenient for the patient to get their medicines from hospital even though clinical responsibility lies with the GP (and vice versa).

The area of outpatient prescribing is currently one of the most contentious because of the financial restrictions and the new NHS initiatives. It is particularly important to clarify who has responsibility for prescribing expensive medicines but in most cases this will lie with the hospital and there will be major cost implications in correcting this.

6. *Patients Own Medicines in Hospital*

Many patients are taking medicines prescribed by their GP on admission to hospital. This is often a source of confusion to hospital doctors and in some cases the therapy is changed to comply with the hospital formulary and the patients' own medicines have been destroyed. In many cases the patient will bring their medicines to hospital all mixed up in a single container and it is difficult to identify the medicines and impossible to guarantee quality. In such circumstances the medicines have to be destroyed. A recent survey in Liverpool showed that the majority of patients brought their medicines into hospital in this way. However, there is an increasing trend for individual packeting of drugs or unit dose dispensing and it will be clear what the identity of the medicines is and that their quality is assured. In such circumstances the medicines should not be destroyed but returned to the patient. In many cases, for patients whose admission to hospital is for a brief period, it is possible to use their own medicines as prescribed by the GP. It makes no sense in these cases to change therapy just to comply with the hospital formulary. If drug therapy is changed, when the patient is discharged from hospital, the hospital doctor must make it clear to the patient and to the general practitioner which medicines should be taken by the patient and how those medicines should be taken.

Conclusions

I have discussed a number of areas of problems that affect the interface between hospital and community prescribing. In general they are due to hospitals offloading costs onto the community and GPs are becoming increasingly resentful of these activities as they come to terms with their own budgeting activities. The answer to these problems is easy to state but difficult to put into practice. Hospitals should prescribe and dispense a greater proportion of medicines they feel are needed for patients, particularly where the clinical responsibility for a patient lies in the hospital sphere. This solution clearly has cost implications for the hospital. Not only will the drug budget need to be increased, but there may need to be an increased establishment of pharmacists to cope with the workload and in a few cases pharmacies in hospital may need structural changes. In the Mersey Region I estimate that the increased costs falling on the hospital sector might be about £4 million per year. However from what I have said, the savings will be considerably greater than this and thus finance would only be needed in the first year. If the system were to work optimally there should be enough flexibility to save more money than the increased expenditure in hospitals. Thus the Regional drug budget would be able to afford the new and expensive medicines recently marketed, and largely cover those that will be introduced in the near future. Since the problem is a national one I believe it needs to be solved nationally and a single infusion of resource should suffice. I am aware that many of these problems only apply in England and Wales since for many years it has been unusual to prescribe for hospital outpatients in Scotland.

Acknowledgements

I am grateful to many friends and colleagues with whom I have discussed these issues over the past few years. However, the responsibility for the views expressed in this chapter are mine alone.

References

1. Ziegler, E. J., Fischer, C. J., Sprung, C. L., Straube, R. C., Sadoff, J. C., Foulke, G. E. *et al.* (1991). Treatment of gram negative bacteremia and septic shock with HA-1A human mono-clonal antibody against endotoxin. *New Engl. J. Med.* **324**, 29–436.
2. Gabriel, R. (1991). Picking up the tab for erythropoetin. *Brit. Med. J.* **302**, 248–249.
3. Cunliffe, W. J., Gray, J. A., MacDonald-Hull, S., Hughes, B. R., Calvert, R. T., Burnside, C. J. *et al.* (1991). Cost effectiveness of isotretinoin. *J. Dermatol. Treat.* **1**, 285–288.
4. Smith, R. (1991). Christie Hospital reports on interleukin 2 controversy. *Brit. Med. J.* **302**, 1041.
5. Anonymous (1989). Local drug formularies – are they worth the effort? *Drug Ther. Bull.* **27**, 13–16.
6. Secretaries of State for Health, Wales, Northern Ireland and Scotland (1989). Working for patients. London, *H.M.S.O.* (Cmnd 555).

Editors' Note

Guidelines (EL(91)127, dated 1 November 1991) were issued by the NHS Management Executive, Department of Health, to Regional General Managers, FHSA General Managers, SHA General Managers and NHS Trust Chief Executives on 'Responsibility for prescribing between hospitals and GPs and are as follows:

Responsibility for Prescribing between Hospitals and GPs

Introduction

1. On 25 February 1987 Sir Leonard Peach, the then acting Chairman of the NHS Management Board, issued guidance on prescribing policy. The guidance indicated that it was for the doctor who had clinical responsibility for a patient to undertake the necessary prescribing. The guidance in the letter ceased to be operational on 1 March 1991 and is superseded by this guidance which, however, preserves its basic principles.

Background

2. The previous guidance referred to cases where hospitals inappropriately transferred prescribing responsibility to GPs. This practice still occurs and causes difficulty to patients, GPs and consultants.

3. With this in mind, and the introduction of indicative prescribing amounts from 1 April 1991, it was important to reconsider the issue of interface prescribing with the aim of providing updated guidance to the NHS. In June 1990, the Department of Health set up a working group of NHS professionals and managers operating prescribing policy day-to-day and charged it with examining current prescribing practices in relation to government health policy. The main issues that needed to be addressed were:

   – **GPs' concerns over taking responsibility for unfamiliar treatment.** GPs were worried about their potential liability for a patient's treatment and there was genuine professional concern over whether it was appropriate for them to take on this prescribing, either wholly or on a shared-care basis;

   – **GPs' concerns over taking additional responsibility for expensive treatment.** With the advent of the indicative prescribing scheme, many GPs were concerned about the effect of out-patient prescribing on their prescribing costs;

   – **consultants' concerns** about prescribing drugs for which there was not budgetary cover;

   – **lack of consultation between professionals over the transfer of prescribing responsibility.** GPs often felt that they had been improperly forced into taking on out-patient prescribing. If they refused, patients may have been denied necessary treatment;

   – patients who are caught in the middle of a professional dispute were worried about the **continuity of their treatment** and the threat that they may be denied treatment, particularly where expensive drugs were involved;

   – **hospitals providing insufficient quantities of drugs on discharge or following an out-patient/casualty visit,** to allow patients time to obtain follow-on treatment from GPs;

- patients having the **additional inconvenience of obtaining prescriptions via their general practitioner**, rather than directly from hospital, immediately after a hospital visit.

4. The deliberations of the Working Group were enhanced by a study* conducted by a research team from St. George's Hospital Medical School.

5. The NHS Management Executive, having considered the helpful views and advice provided by the Working Group, has produced the following guidance to address the above concerns. The guidance re-affirms the policy that prescribing responsibility will continue to be based on clinical responsibility. This is good medical practice and is in the best interests of the patient.

The Indicative Prescribing Scheme

6. The guidance given below sets out the basis on which prescribing responsibility should be determined and, where appropriate, transferred. General practitioners should note that the operation of the indicative prescribing scheme does not in any way inhibit them financially from accepting prescribing responsibility under these guidelines.

Clinical Responsibility and the Prescription of Drugs

General Principles

7. When clinical, and therefore prescribing, responsibility for a patient is transferred from hospital to GP, it is of the utmost importance that the GP has full confidence to prescribe the necessary drugs. It is, therefore, essential that a transfer involving drug therapies with which GPs would not normally be familiar should not take place without *full* local agreement and the dissemination of sufficient information to individual GPs. When drawing up protocols or where there is a professional disagreement over who should prescribe, it may be necessary for local discussion to take place between DHAs, hospital managers and medical staff, FHSAs and the relevant LMC as a prelude to establishing agreement with individual GPs. A GP of course is only obliged to provide treatment consistent with the terms of service for GPs set out in the NHS (GMPS) Regulations.

8. Legal responsibility for prescribing lies with the doctor who signs the prescription.

9. When a GP takes responsibility for prescribing or dispensing drugs which have not normally been dispensed in the community, there should be liaison between the transferring hospital and the community pharmacists to ensure a continuity of supply of the drug.

In-patients

10. Hospital consultants have full clinical responsibility for in-patients under their care, as well as responsibility for all drugs prescribed to them.

11. When a patient is discharged from hospital, sufficient drugs and dressings should normally be prescribed by the hospital and dispensed by the hospital pharmacy, where possible, for a minimum of 7 days after discharge unless the drugs are not required for so long a period. The GP, to whose care the patient is being transferred, should receive notification *in adequate time* of the patient's diagnosis and drug therapy so that any on-going treatment can be maintained. In the event that information about the patient cannot be transferred from hospital to GP within the timescale, drugs should be prescribed by the hospital for as long a period as necessary.

Patients Attending Accident and Emergency

12. Patients attending an Accident and Emergency unit should also receive a supply of drugs from the hospital for 7 days, or less if drugs are not required for that length of time. Any appropriate prescribing after that period will then rest with the GP responsible for the patient's continuing care.

---

* Prescribing at the Hospital/General Practice Inferface: Current Hospital Dispensing Policies in England and their impact on Hospital Chief Pharmacists, General Practitioners, Hospital Consultants and Community Pharmacists – Anderson, Preeling, Rafferty, Sibbald, Wilkie, April 1991.

Out-patients

13. Consultants have full responsibility for prescribing drugs and dressings for specific treatments administered in hospital out-patient clinics.

14. Subject to paragraph 15, where a consultant feels that he or she should initiate immediate treatment to an out-patient, drugs should normally be prescribed for the patient by the hospital and dispensed, where possible, by the hospital pharmacy for not less than 14 days. In other instances the consultant may request that the GP consider initiating or continuing treatment. The consultant should give the GP notification *in adequate time* of the patient's diagnosis and drug therapy so that any on-going treatment can be maintained. In the event that information about the patient cannot be transferred from hospital to GP within the timescale, drugs should be prescribed by the consultant for as long a period as necessary.

Shared Care

15. When a consultant considers a patient's condition is stable, he may seek the agreement of the GP concerned to share care. In proposing a shared care arrangement, a consultant may advise the general practitioner which medicine to prescribe. Where a new, or rarely prescribed, medicine is being recommended, its dosage and administration must be specified by the consultant so that the GP is properly informed and can monitor treatment and adjust the dose if necessary. In addition, when a treatment is not licensed for a particular indication, then full justification for the use of the drug should be given by the consultant to the GP. Provision of a protocol for treatment should normally be provided. Where a hospital drug formulary is in operation and a recommended treatment is not included, the GP must be informed that this is the case and given the option of prescribing alternatives.

Where Responsibility for Prescribing Should Remain with Consultants

16. Occasions will arise when responsibility for prescribing for a patient, who is otherwise under the care of his or her GP, will more appropriately rest with a consultant, for example where:
    - drugs are undergoing or included in a hospital based clinical trial;
    - the consultant considers that only he is able to monitor the patient's response to medication because, for example, of the need for specialised investigations;
    - drugs or appliances are only available through hospitals or where there are supply problems.

Role of Regional Health Authorities (RHAs)

17. RHAs are well placed to encourage and facilitate developments which better integrate the care provided and ensure a smooth transition of patients from hospital to GP and vice versa. Their responsibility is to ensure that local prescribing policies are compatible with this guidance and that patient care is 'seamless'.

18. In particular, RHAs should further stimulate the representation of joint primary and secondary care interests through debate in Drug and Therapeutics Committees, and facilitate development of treatment protocols in which GPs, consultants and other appropriate health care professionals can locally agree how certain treatments should be handled.

19. FHSA, via their Medical Advisers, in co-operation with hospital consultants, should ensure that GPs are sufficiently informed on new and/or unfamiliar drugs and the related local prescribing policies. Regional Pharmaceutical Officers (RPhOs), through their drug information services, are able to provide support. Telephone numbers are given in the British National Formulary (BNF).

Contracting and the Reforms

20. With the inception of the NHS reforms from 1 April, the Department of Health will be encouraging RHAs, through the contracting system, to identify the extent of local hospital drug provision and to ensure that it is consistent, or made consistent, with these guidelines. Specifying local hospitals' drug provision responsibilities in contracts should lead to a more effective and efficient targeting of the necessary resources towards the provision of hospital drugs. RHAs should ensure that this objective is pursued as vigorously as possible, in the interests of patient care.

Index